CHURCHILL'S POCKETBOOK OF
Oncology

Lester Barr
ChM FRCS
Consultant Surgeon,
University Hospitals of South Manchester
and Christie Hospital, Manchester, UK

Richard Cowan
MD MRCP FRCR
Consultant Clinical Oncologist,
Christie Hospital, Manchester, UK

Marianne Nicolson
MD FRCP
Consultant Medical Oncologist,
Aberdeen Royal Hospitals Trust
Aberdeen, UK

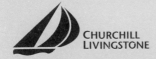

**CHURCHILL
LIVINGSTONE**

NEW YORK EDINBURGH LONDON MADRID
MELBOURNE SAN FRANCISCO AND TOKYO 1997

CHURCHILL LIVINGSTONE
Medical Division of Pearson Professional Limited

Distributed in the United States of America by
Churchill Livingstone Inc., 650 Avenue of the
Americas, New York, N.Y. 10011, and by associated
companies, branches and representatives throughout
the world.

First published 1997

Standard Edition ISBN 0 443 05102 X

International Student Edition first published 1997
International Student Edition ISBN 0 443 05689 7

British Library Cataloguing in Publication Data
A catalogue record for this book is available from
the British Library.

Library of Congress Cataloging in Publication Data
A catalog record for this book is available from
the Library of Congress.

Medical knowledge is constantly changing. As new
information becomes available, changes in treatment,
procedures, equipment and the use of drugs become
necessary. The authors and the publishers have, as
far as it is possible, taken care to ensure that the
information given in the text is accurate and up to
date. However, readers are strongly advised to
confirm that the information, especially with regard
to drug usage, complies with current legislation and
standards of practice.

The
publisher's
policy is to use
**paper manufactured
from sustainable forests**

Produced by Longman Singapore Publishers Pte Ltd
Printed in Singapore

Contents

4. Managing specific tumours

5. Appendices

Abbreviations

ACE	angiotensin-converting enzyme	COAD	chronic obstructive airways disease
ACTH	adrenocorticotrophic hormone	CSF	cerebrospinal fluid
ADH	antidiuretic hormone	CT	computerised tomography
AF	atrial fibrillation	CVP	central venous pressure
AFP	alpha fetoprotein (tumour marker for hepatic and germ cell tumours)	CXR	chest X-ray
		d	day (s)
		D&C	dilatation and curettage
AIDS	autoimmune deficiency syndrome	DCIS	ductal carcinoma in-situ
		DIC	disseminated intravascular coagulation
ALL	acute lymphoblastic leukaemia	DNA	deoxyribonucleic acid
AML	acute myeloblastic leukaemia	DVT	deep venous thrombosis
		EBV	Epstein Barr virus
AXR	abdominal X-ray	ECG	electrocardiogram
bHCG	human chorionic gonadotrophin	EDTA	ethylene diamine tetra acetate (a method of calculating GFR)
BCG	Bacille Calmette Guérin	ENT	ear, nose and throat
BP	blood pressure	ERCP	endoscopic retrograde cholangiopancreatography
BPH	benign prostatic hypertrophy	ESR	erythrocyte sedimentation rate
BSO	bilateral salpingo-oophorectomy	EUA	examination under anaesthetic
CA19.9	tumour marker for pancreatic cancer	FBC	full blood count
CA125	tumour marker for ovarian cancer	FNAC	fine needle aspirate cytology
CEA	carcinoembryonic antigen (tumour marker for colon cancer)	g	grams
		gCSF	granulocyte colony stimulating factor
CIN	cervical intra-epithelial neoplasia	GA	general anaesthetic
Cl	chloride ion	GI	gastrointestinal
CLL	chronic lymphatic leukaemia	GFR	glomerular filtration rate
		GP	general practitioner
CMV	cytomegalovirus	GRH	gonadotrophin releasing hormone
CML	chronic myeloid leukaemia	GVHD	graft versus host disease

Preface

Oncology must be one of the most exciting and rewarding areas of medicine to be involved in! It is a rapidly changing field, with a close interface between clinical practice and a huge scientific research effort. It involves team work between surgeons, oncologists, palliative care and nurse specialists. The day to day management of oncology patients is emotionally as well as intellectually challenging. The primary aim is of course to cure, but when this is not possible difficult decisions must be made with the patient about quality of life issues.

The aim of this book is to be a concise summary of current diagnostic and therapeutic techniques across a broad range of oncological problems, and we hope that it will appeal to doctors, nurses, allied health professionals and members of the public alike.

L. B.   1997
R. C.
M. N.

C
C
CE
CIN
C
CLL
CMV
CML

h	hour
H+	hydrogen ion
5HIAA	5 hydroxyindole acetic acid
HIV	human immunodeficiency virus
HRT	hormone replacement therapy
5HT	5 hydroxy tryptamine
HLA	human leucocyte antigen
IA	intra-arterial
ICP	intracranial pressure
IM	intramuscular
IT	intrathecal
IU	international units
IV	intravenous
IVC	inferior vena cava
IVU	intravenous urogram
K+	potassium ion
l	litre
L	lumbar
LCIS	lobular carcinoma in situ
LD	latissimus dorsi
LDH	lactate dehydrogenase
LP	lumbar puncture
LVEF	left ventricular ejection fraction
MEN	multiple endocrine neoplasia syndrome
MESNA	sodium 2-mercaptoethanesulphonate
MI	myocardial infarction
MR (I)	magnetic resonance (imaging)
MTD	maximum tolerated dose
Na+	sodium ion
NG	nasogastric
NHL	non-Hodgkin's lymphoma
NSAID	non-steroidal anti-inflammatory drug
NSCLC	non-small cell lung cancer
OPG	orthopantomogram
pCO$_2$	carbon dioxide tension
pO$_2$	oxygen tension
PE	pulmonary embolism
PEG	percutaneous endoscopic gastrostomy
PP	paraprotein
PSA	prostatic surface antigen (tumour marker)
PTC	percutaneous transhepatic cholangiogram
PTH	parathyroid hormone
PUO	pyrexia of unknown origin
QDS	four times daily
RPLND	retroperitoneal lymph node dissection
SAIDH	syndrome of inappropriate ADH
SCC	squamous cell carcinoma
SCLC	small cell lung cancer
SVC (O)	superior vena cava (obstruction)
T	thoracic
TAH	total abdominal hysterectomy
TCC	transitional cell carcinoma
TDS	three times daily
TENS	transcutaneous electrical nerve stimulation
TNM	tumour, nodes metastases staging system
TNS	transcutaneous nerve stimulation
TNF	tumour necrosis factor
TRAM	transverse rectus abdominis myocutaneous
TUR	transurethral resection
TVU	transvaginal ultrasound
U&Es	urea and electrolytes
VAIN	vaginal intraepithelial neoplasia

Oncological terms

Apoptosis Programmed cell death or the mechanism by which chemotherapy and irradiation cause tumour cells to die.

Doubling time Time taken for the tumour to double in size, e.g. 30 days in SCLC, 129 days in NSCLC.

Median survival Time following diagnosis by which 50% of patients have died.

Therapeutic ratio Quotient of response over toxicity.

Therapeutic window Difference between the optimum response and unacceptable toxicity; may be 'narrow' or 'wide'.

Objective response Measured clinical or radiological shrinkage of tumour (see WHO criteria).

Symptomatic response Measured improvement in patient's symptoms / performance status.

Quality of life Measurement through validated questionnaires of various parameters including symptoms, mood, sociabliity, etc.

Adjuvant 'Back-up' treatment with chemotherapy or radiotherapy following an apparently curative resection of tumour.

Neoadjuvant Preoperative chemo- or radiotherapy given to shrink the primary tumour, facilitate surgery and possibly to treat unmeasurable micrometastases.

Palliative Treatment given to improve symptoms and possibly to increase life expectancy without prospect of cure.

Progression free survival Duration of response to treatment where no measurable increase in tumour size is seen.

Minimal residual disease Situation post maximum debulking of tumour where it is known that there is still a small amount of tumour left behind.

Tumour flare Increase in tumour-related symptoms, e.g. bone pain, seen especially in patients with advanced breast or prostate cancer who have been started on hormonal therapy; usually occurs within the first month of therapy.

Relapse Recurrence of tumour following a response to therapy.

Remission Shrinkage of tumour, sometimes so that none can be measured clinically, radiologically or on blood tests following treatment. For definition of complete and partial remission, see page 180 (WHO response criteria).

Staging Evaluation of extent of tumour using clinical, radiological and surgical (e.g. laparoscopy) techniques.

MANAGING A PATIENT WITH CANCER

COMMUNICATION AND COUNSELLING

Effective communication rarely takes place during a doctor's or nurse's monologue, however brilliant. You need to listen as well as to speak in order to ascertain the patient's needs and level of understanding.

Guidelines for effective communication

- Put the disease into its psychological and social context (e.g. 'what concerns you most about your illness?'). Not only is this good 'holistic' medicine, but it also makes practical sense since it gives you cues as to the issues concerning prognosis or treatment that need to be discussed. Ask if the patient would like a partner or friend to be present at the interview.
- Ask what the patient has already been told and establish the level of understanding for further discussion.
- Avoid jargon (e.g. 'prognosis', 'adjuvant').
- Avoid euphemisms (e.g. 'misbehaving cells' rather than the more painful but honest explanation of cancer).
- Avoid closed questions (i.e. those which are answered simply by yes or no). Open-ended questions give the patient an opportunity to bring up unresolved issues.
- Involve the patient in decision making. Few desire complete autonomy, but most wish to have some relevant background information and to feel that they are still 'in control'.
- Introduce diagnostic procedures and consent to treatment with brief explanations. Give the patient time to ask questions.
- Ask the patient for feedback with open questions (e.g. 'Tell me what you can remember of the things I've said'), rather than closed questions (e.g. 'Do you understand?').

Witholding information: 'Please don't tell him'

Protective relatives may request that the diagnosis be withheld from a patient. You should explain that:

- The information about test results etc. is primarily the property of the patient.
- You will respond to the patient's questions with honest answers.
- You will not force unrequested information on the patient.
- Most patients realise the gravity of the situation from non-verbal communication, and a conspiracy of silence often increases their sense of isolation from family members at a time when they most need closeness and warmth.

The bad news interview

Initial diagnosis

This is made easier if you have prepared the patient beforehand, e.g. 'I'll have the results of your tests tomorrow, when I'll come to see you again. Perhaps you'd find it helpful to have a friend or relative with you'. Avoid delay and do not use the telephone or the formal ward round. Find a quiet room and sit so you are all at eye level, including the supporting relative or friend. Begin with a preliminary warning, e.g. 'I am sorry to say that I have bad news', and break the news sympathetically, making use of the Guidelines above. Explain treatment strategy simply and leave the patient with a hopeful (but realistic) message. Give opportunity for a further meeting, when treatment can be explained and questions answered in more detail. Involve other professionals (e.g. the GP or a nurse counsellor. Give written information to the patient, and suggest they write down any questions that may occur to them after this meeting for discussion next time.

Recurrence

The diagnosis of recurrent disease can be as devastating as the initial diagnosis of cancer, or even more so. Fear of dying, of terminal illness and suffering, fears for the family, feelings of self-pity and self-doubt and disillusionment with the medical profession, are all common and may need to be explored and dealt with. Don't be tempted to give false reassurances that all will be well if this is not the case; be honest and explain the treatment strategies available and the likelihood of a temporary or long-term remission or cure.

Withdrawing active anticancer treatment

Many patients will come to the point where active intervention with surgery, radiotherapy or chemotherapy is no longer appropriate because cure is no longer a possibility. This needs to be discussed honestly with your patient, but give reassurances about the effectiveness of modern pain control (see pp. 58–60) and explain about palliative care (see p. 15). The decision not to resuscitate in the event of cardio-respiratory arrest on the ward should be taken by the appropriate consultant and not by a more junior member of the medical team, and only after sensitive discussion with the patient or with their relatives.

Using nurse counsellors

Many patients value the care offered by a nurse counsellor. In her absence, a senior nurse or outpatient nurse may assume the role. It is a good idea for her to be present at a 'bad news' interview as she will provide continuity of care and support throughout treatment and after discharge. This does not relieve the doctor of the responsibility for making and discussing treatment decisions or in addressing significant psychological problems.

The angry relative

You may be asked to see an 'angry relative'. Anger often betrays an underlying anxiety or fear, or it can be used as a method of gaining attention or action when a relative considers the degree of communication by the medical team to have been inadequate previously. The following tactics may be useful:

- Don't respond to anger with anger or to aggression with aggression.
- Calm the situation down by being pleasant and expressing a desire to help.
- Point out that you also want the very best for the patient concerned and are therefore 'on the same side' as the angry relative.
- Don't be afraid to apologise if the angry relative has a legitimate complaint.
- Often anger may surround a simple misunderstanding which can easily be cleared up.
- If you are worried about physical aggression, take someone else with you and meet in a non-enclosed public area.
- Keep an accurate, dated, written report of your conversation.

PRINCIPLES OF SURGERY

Diagnosis and management

About 80% of patients with a suspected tumour are referred first to a surgeon. With the current emphasis in diagnosis and management of cancer on a team approach, the surgical oncologist requires a keen awareness of alternative non-surgical treatment strategies, of the role of adjuvant and neoadjuvant therapies and of the need for close collaboration in treatment protocols and clinical trials with his radiotherapy and medical oncology colleagues.

Biopsy

A cytological diagnosis of malignancy following a smear or fine needle aspirate may be sufficient to allow therapeutic intervention, but more usually a needle core biopsy or an open surgical biopsy is required before embarking on a major treatment programme. There are some important rules:

- The tissue must be representative of the whole lesion
  — avoid areas of necrosis or haemorrhage
  — take multiple endoscopic or needle biopsies to avoid false negative
  — make every effort to obtain adequate tissue at the first attempt.
- The biopsy should not be crushed or charred during the operation.
- Biopsies from skin or mucosal surfaces should include the junction between normal and abnormal tissues.
- Avoid implantation of cells into adjacent healthy tissues when a deep lesion is biopsied, e.g. wound drains are not inserted through a separate stab incision.

- The biopsy incision should not compromise any possible subsequent definitive surgery, e.g. biopsy incisions on the limbs should be vertically orientated rather than horizontal.
- The pathologist must be supplied with accurate clinical data.

Staging

Surgery may be required to provide information on disease stage if this will influence decisions regarding adjuvant therapies. CT scan assessment and the increasing role of chemotherapy, e.g. for patients with Hodgkin's disease, has removed the need for staging laparotomy in many cases. Axillary dissection remains important in breast cancer, since axillary node status may determine whether or not a woman receives adjuvant cytotoxic chemotherapy. Laparoscopic staging of pelvic lymph node involvement for carcinoma of the bladder and prostate is often more accurate than CT staging.

Curative resection

Curative resection should be attempted in patients assessed preoperatively as having:

- no metastases
- a lesion that is technically resectable with a margin of healthy surrounding tissue.

The principles are:

- 'En-bloc' dissection—resection of all of the involved tissues, together with any regional lymph nodes that may be at risk, without breaching any plane that may contain tumour.
- Cosmetic and functional considerations.

Examples of curative resection

'En-bloc' dissection
- Locally advanced carcinoma of the colon may require resection of a portion of abdominal wall and/or dome of bladder together with the involved bowel.
- In carcinoma of the rectum, lateral spread into pelvic lymph nodes is more important than vertical spread through the bowel wall; a careful pelvic node dissection is imperative whereas a margin of 3 cm distal to the palpable edge of tumour in the rectal wall may be sufficient to preserve the anal sphincters while preventing local recurrence.
- Carcinoma of the oesophagus requires proximal and distal margins of excision of 10 cm because of the propensity for submucosal spread along the oesophageal wall.

Cosmetic and functional considerations
- The margin of clearance around a cutaneous malignant melanoma < 2 mm in depth does not need to exceed 1 cm, thus avoiding mutilating scars.

Laparoscopic surgery

The place of laparoscopy in oncology is expanding as techniques and procedures are developed. Of particular importance are:

- assessing operability in cancer of the stomach and lower oesophagus
- palliative bypass surgery, e.g. gastroenterostomy
- staging of bladder and prostate cancer.

Palliation

Surgery is often justified in the face of incurable advanced disease, where the intention is palliative rather than to prolong survival.

Examples of palliative surgery

- Laparotomy to resect, bypass or defunction an obstructing malignant process in a hollow organ, e.g. ureter, stomach, small or large bowel
- Stenting of obstructed ureter at cystoscopy by cannulation with a 'double-J' catheter
- 'Toilet' procedure, e.g. simple mastectomy or amputation of a limb, for fungating tumours
- Lymph node dissection for breast cancer to prevent unpleasant, uncontrolled nodal disease

---

Debulking surgery

There are theoretical reasons for believing that a reduction in the cancer cell burden prior to commencing chemotherapy can increase the likelihood of complete remission. This has led to debulking surgery becoming standard practice in the initial management of carcinoma of the ovary.

There is evidence to show that patients with carcinoma of the ovary treated by total abdominal hysterectomy with bilateral salpingo-oophorectomy and omentectomy, in which no macroscopic disease is left behind, achieve better results than those treated by a smaller operative procedure.

Debulking surgery may also be useful as a palliative measure for large-volume tumours that are causing pressure symptoms, e.g. a large retroperitoneal sarcoma.

Second-look laparotomy

There was a vogue in the 1960s and 1970s for second-look laparotomy in patients who had previously undergone 'curative' resection for carcinoma of the colon. The decision to operate was based on a rise in serum CEA levels or recurrent symptoms. Occasionally a second chance at cure for local recurrence or solitary liver metastasis was achieved, but for most patients recurrent disease proved to be surgically incurable. CEA is not sufficiently accurate as a serum marker to be used in this way. Nevertheless, some patients undoubtedly benefit from a second attempt at cure by radical surgery when local recurrence is discovered and quantified by modern imaging techniques.

In cancer of the ovary, it has been common practice to carry out second-look laparotomy to assess the response to chemotherapy, but lack of impact on survival has made this procedure less common in the UK.

Metastasectomy

Metastasectomy is one of the commonest indications for lung resection and liver resection in the developed world. Prolonged survival may be seen following pulmonary resection for:

- metastatic osteogenic sarcoma
- soft-tissue sarcoma
- occasionally, carcinoma (e.g. renal, colorectal).

Liver resection for metastatic colorectal cancer has not been investigated by randomized trials, but does result in long-term 'cure' for some patients. The best results are achieved in patients with:

- either a solitary metastasis, or
- fewer than four lesions, all of which must be surgically resectable with clear margins.

Reconstruction

Plastic and reconstructive surgery has made an enormous impact in the management of head and neck cancers and in limb sarcomas in recent years, through the use of pedicled and free flaps, often in combination with recent improvements in prosthetics. For breast cancer, several techniques for breast and nipple reconstruction have been described. The most commonly used are:

- latissimus dorsi (LD) flap
- transverse rectus abdominis myocutaneous (TRAM) flap.

Intra-arterial chemotherapy

A surgically placed intra-arterial catheter for regional perfusion of an organ or tissue with cytotoxic drugs produces an enhanced therapeutic/toxic ratio, e.g. isolated limb perfusion with high-dose melphalan for malignant melanoma with metastases confined to one limb, by which dramatic responses can be achieved. In some centres hepatic artery infusional chemotherapy gives better response rates than intravenous chemotherapy, although its impact on overall survival is less certain since most patients die of extrahepatic disease. Complications include:

- hepatitis
- pain
- catheter displacement
- infection.

PRINCIPLES OF RADIOTHERAPY

Mechanism of action

Ionising radiation is a highly potent cytotoxic agent. It reacts with both normal and malignant cells to induce intracellular chemical reactions with the production of very short half life, highly ionised molecules termed *free radicals*. Free radicals damage cellular DNA by disrupting the disulphide bonds within the double helix, causing irreversible damage (double strand breaks), or reversible damage (single strand breaks). The cell may then continue to perform its normal metabolic activities, and the DNA damage may only become manifest when the cell comes to divide. Disruption or prevention of malignant cell division leads to disruption or cessation of tumour growth.

Normal cells have a better capacity for repairing sublethal radiation damage than cancer cells. This differential repair capacity is exploited in radiotherapy.

Fractionation of radiotherapy

Radiation cell killing is conventionally expressed in terms of a cell survival curve (Fig. 1.1) which has two components. The initial curving region (shoulder) represents the reversible DNA damage which can be manipulated to improve the therapeutic ratio while the exponential region reflects the irreversible DNA damage. By dividing the total dose of administered radiation into equal size fractions one can change the shape of the cell survival curve. Fig. 1.2 shows that fractionated radiotherapy causes a lower cell kill compared with an identical total dose of radiation given as a single exposure. Fractionation enhances the therapeutic ratio because of the difference in the shape of the shoulder between malignant cells and normal tissue. The ideal interval between fractions of radiotherapy should be sufficient to allow maximum repair of sublethally damaged normal tissue, yet short enough to limit malignant cell repair and repopulation (Fig. 1.3).

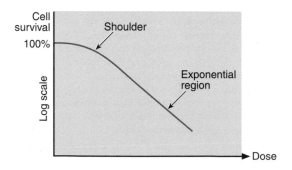

Fig. 1.1 Fractionation of radiotherapy: cell survival curve.

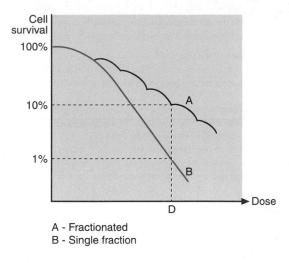

A - Fractionated
B - Single fraction

Fig. 1.2 Fractionation of radiotherapy. Cell kill compared with single exposure radiation.

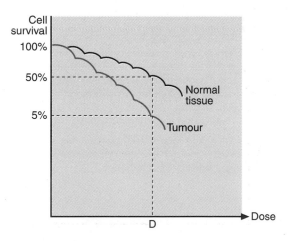

Fig. 1.3 Ideal interval between fractions of radiation.

...tering radiotherapy

There are different methods of administering radiotherapy which allow the precise delivery of ionizing radiation to be delivered to the tumour.

- External beam therapy (*teletherapy*)
  — *kilovoltage therapy*—lower-energy radiation produced by an X-ray source (e.g. for treatment of superficial skin lesions such as basal cell carcinomas)
  — *megavoltage therapy*—high-energy radiation produced by a gamma-emitting source ($Cobalt^{60}$ or $Caesium^{137}$), or more commonly by a linear accelerator (suitable for deep-seated tumours).
- *Brachytherapy*—ionising radiation emitted from a sealed source which is placed in close proximity to the tumour (e.g. intracavitary treatment of carcinoma of the uterine cervix, or implants with iridium wire or caesium needles).

These methods of administration allow us to precribe a precise dose of cytotoxic radiation to be delivered to the tumour.

Determining dosage

When radiotherapy is given with curative intent, the maximum dose is administered up to the limit of 'acceptable' normal tissue damage using optimal fractionation. This dose will be influenced by:

- the radiosensitivity of the tumour (lymphomas are more sensitive than carcinomas)
- the radiosensitivity of the critical normal tissue within the radiation field (e.g. spinal cord)
- the volume of normal tissue unavoidably irradiated.

The art of radiotherapy is to minimize the volume of normal tissue irradiated yet to ensure that the radiation field encompasses the target volume (tumour ± regional lymph nodes) with an adequate margin. Our ability to do this has been enhanced by improved tumour imaging and the capacity for accurate field shaping.

Radiotherapy may be administered with radical or palliative intent.

- Radical—maximum dose administered with 'acceptable' toxicity.
- Palliative—total dose is not so important in symptom relief; emphasis must be on minimizing side-effects of radiation.

PRINCIPLES OF CHEMOTHERAPY

The aim of chemotherapy is not only to kill or shrink the primary tumour but also to kill metastasized cells. In order to understand the theory behind the mechanisms of action of the different chemotherapeutic agents it is necessary to understand the pathophysiology of tumour cells.

Tumour growth

The human body contains about 5×10^{13} cells. Cancer is believed to arise when one of these escapes normal growth control mechanisms. Only when there is a mass of 10^9 cells (1 g) will a tumour become clinically detectable. Obviously, most tumours are much larger than this when they are diagnosed, and in addition there may have been spread of the primary tumour to produce metastatic (secondary) lesions elsewhere in the body.

There are four stages in the cell cycle: G1, initial resting phase; S, synthetic phase during which the DNA duplicates; G2, second resting (premitotic) phase; and M, cell division during which mitosis takes place (Fig. 1.4).

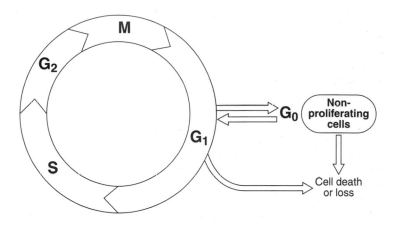

Proliferating cells ('growth fraction')

M	= mitosis
G₁, G₂	= gap
S	= DNA synthesis

Fig. 1.4 Model of a tumour cell population.

The cell cycle time of 90% of human tumour cells is 15–120 h, with an average of 48 h. Even within the same tumour mass there may be significant variation of the duration of the cell cycle which has implications both for tumour growth and for treatment. Those cells which are not actively dividing within the cycle are said to be in the resting or G0 phase. At any time cells may re-enter the cycle and have the capacity for growth. The ratio of tumour cells cycling to total number of cells in the tumour is called the 'growth fraction'. Some rapidly growing tumours, e.g. leukaemias and lymphomas, will have a growth fraction of 90%, whereas for carcinomas and sarcomas the number may be as low as 10%.

The reason for the uncontrolled proliferation of a tumour is not that its cell cycle is more rapid than that of normal cells—it may be much slower—but the control of growth is lost, with division occurring even when it is not necessary to replace dead cells. Tumour cells also lose contact inhibition, so pile on top of each other, allowing a steady increase in tumour size at the expense of normal tissue. The rapid division of cells may produce varying types of cell (a heterogeneous population), some of which may demonstrate different capacities for survival. Some cells may thrive in a relatively hypoxic environment while others may have varying sensitivities to a particular chemotherapeutic agent.

Tumour cells may be lost by exfoliation, especially common in GI tumours, or by outgrowing their blood supply, rendering the centre of the tumour necrotic and non-viable. Some tumour cells will be fatally flawed because of a genetic defect and will die. Others may travel via the lymphatic or haematogenous route and implant elsewhere, resulting in metastatic disease if the secondary tumour can stimulate synthesis of its own blood system through the secretion of angiogenesis factors.

Depending on the cell cycle time, the growth fraction and the rate of cell loss, the tumour doubling time is established. In haematological tumours the doubling time may be exponential (i.e. there is a proportional increase in size with unit time), but in a solid tumour it appears that the tumour growth rate slows as the tumour enlarges. The progressive decrease in rate of growth is termed Gompertzian growth (described in 1825 by the English mathematician, Benjamin Gompertz) and is believed to be related mainly to the relative hypoxia of those cells which lie furthest from the nutritional source (blood supply).

Tumours curable by chemotherapy

Childhood ALL	Choriocarcinoma
Hodgkin's disease	Ovarian cancer
Lymphoma (some)	Wilm's tumour
Germ cell testicular tumours	Embryonal rhabdomyosarcoma
Adult AML	Ewing's sarcoma

Types of chemotherapy

The common chemotherapies can be divided into the following classes according to their chemistry or mode of action:

- alkylating agents
- antimetabolites
- vinca alkaloids
- antimitotic antibiotics
- others.

Alkylating agents Contain an alkyl group (analiphatic hydrocarbon with a hydrogen missing) which allows them to form covalent bonds with other molecules, specifically at the cross-link on the DNA helix, thus preventing the separation of the two strands during DNA replication. The alkylating agents also attach to free guanine bases on separated DNA strands and prevent their acting as templates for new DNA formation.

Antimetabolites Have a similar chemical structure to essential metabolites which are required by the cell prior to cell division. The antimetabolites may be incorporated into the new nuclear material or may combine irreversibly with vital enzymes to inhibit division of the cells. Mechanisms of action include antagonism to folic acid (e.g. methotrexate) or purine (e.g. 6-mercaptopurine, 6-thioguanine), inhibition of thymidylate synthase (e.g. 5-fluorouracil) or DNA polymerase (e.g. cytosine arabinoside) and incorporation of a fluoridated nucleoside in place of the normal nucleoside (e.g. 5-fluorouracil instead of uracil in RNA).

Vinca alkaloids Metaphase arrest agents, derived from the periwinkle plant *Vinca rosea*. They bind to tubuli, blocking microtubule formation and therefore cell spindle formation which is essential for the metaphase stage of mitosis.

Antimitotic antibiotics May be divided into anthracyclines and non-anthracyclines. Their mode of action is not certain but includes:

- intercalation—inhibiting DNA and RNA synthesis
- membrane binding—increasing cell membrane permeability to various ions
- free radical formation—disrupting the DNA chain and preventing mitosis
- metal ion chelation—resulting in cytotoxic compounds
- alkylation—blocking DNA replication.

Taxanes Taxol and taxotere are relatively new first- and second-generation agents which act by spindle promotion. Their activity against breast and ovarian cancers is established, but their individual role in oncology is yet to be determined.

Other classes
Non-classical alkylating agents Cisplatin and carboplatin are two commonly used platinum-based drugs which block DNA replication by forming intra- and interstrand cross-links on the DNA helix. Dacarbazine (DTIC) is a purine analogue which may, following metabolism, act like an alkylating agent. Procarbazine is an analogue of the monoamine oxidase inhibitors. It may act by alkylation.

Anthracenediones Mitozantrone has a structure similar to the anthracyclines. It acts by DNA intercalation but causes less free radical formation, which reduces its cardiotoxicity.

Epidophyllotoxins Etoposide is a semisynthetic analogue of podophyllotoxin. Its mode of action is not completely understood, but it is thought that it arrests DNA replication in the premitotic phase.

Hydroxyurea Analogue of urea, first synthesized 100 years ago. It inhibits ribonucleotide reductase and prevents DNA synthesis.

Combination chemotherapy
It is important to establish the single agent activity for a drug before using it in combined therapy. Combination regimens are commonly known by the first letters of the drugs included, for example adriamycin, cyclophosphamide and etoposide: ACE.

The rationale for combination chemotherapy is twofold:

- Different drugs exert their effect through different mechanisms and at different stages of the cell cycle, thus the aim is to maximize the number and types of cancer cells killed with each treatment cycle. Some anticancer drugs may be synergistic (e.g. cisplatin and 5-fluorouracil), which makes combination therapy even more attractive.
- Combining drugs decreases the chance of drug resistance developing in the tumour, which otherwise has a great capacity for adapting to increase its survival potential.

Consideration of the individual drug toxicities is essential when combining chemotherapies into a regimen since severe morbidity or even mortality for the patient may result from the combination of drugs whose main side-effect is, for example, nephrotoxicity.

Dosing frequency
Chemotherapy is delivered intermittently rather than at a constant low dose, to exploit the fact that malignant cells have a less effective repair capacity than normal cells. The optimum dosing will achieve maximum tumour cell kill, with the next treatment cycle given when normal stem cells have had adequate time to recover from the first—too soon and the normal cell

population will suffer unacceptable toxicity; too late and the tumour will be allowed to recover to its pretreatment size or expand. Intermittent therapy also allows the immune function time to recover and therefore to maintain its role in tumour surveillance.

Toxicity of chemotherapy

Cancer patients are often much more reluctant to receive chemotherapy than surgery or radiotherapy. The main reason for this is the perceived severity of toxic side-effects of chemotherapy. To a great extent, the most common side-effects can now be alleviated, and it is possible to reassure patients that appropriate remedies are available. It is important that patients are issued with a typed information sheet detailing the expected side-effects of treatment and are given the opportunity to ask questions and discuss their anxieties before they start chemotherapy. They should be informed whom to contact and when in the event of toxicity. For details on the main toxicities and their management, refer to Section 3.

Calculation of drug dose

In most cases chemotherapy is delivered in a dose which is calculated from the weight and height of the patient, expressed as x mg/m^2 (see Appendix, p. 181). The duration of time for which the drug remains in the body will depend on the rate of metabolism and of clearance. According to the route of clearance there may be a formula to calculate the correct dose. It is important to note that if a drug is metabolized in the liver (e.g. doxorubicin), it will be around for longer and this may increase its toxicity to normal cells. Equally, where the drug is cleared through the kidneys (e.g. cisplatin), it is important to establish the renal function by measuring creatinine clearance or performing a ^{51}Cr-EDTA to measure glomerular filtration.

PALLIATIVE CARE

For cancer patients who come to the point where there is no longer any potential for cure, the emphasis of treatment may need to shift from prolongation of survival to improving the quality of the remaining length of life. In this situation the toxicity of therapeutic intervention needs to be carefully considered. There are three important aspects to palliative care:

- symptom control
- addressing psychosocial concerns
- the organization of care within the community.

Symptom control

The major topics concerning symptom control are discussed in detail in Sections 2 and 3—pain management, nausea and vomiting, constipation, etc. The most effective control may be achieved by surgery (e.g. intestinal obstruction), radiotherapy (e.g. brain metastases) or chemotherapy (e.g. liver metastases), depending on the symptom, but the patient should usually be made aware of the lack of curative intent before embarking on treatment that may in the short term add to their morbidity.

Psychosocial concerns

The following should be considered:

- communication within the family (pp. 2–4)
- helping the patient cope with increasing disability
- looking for evidence of depressive illness, and
- involvement of other professionals such as a counsellor.

Screening for depression

You will need to distinguish between understandable *sadness* during terminal illness and *clinical depression*. Biological symptoms of depression (e.g. anorexia, weight loss) are difficult to interpret in cancer patients, but early morning waking with morbid thoughts are good indicators of depression. A combination of an antidepressant (e.g. dothiepin) with increased psychological support is ideal treatment.

Symptoms of depression
Sleep (early morning waking)
Appetite (poor)
Weight (loss)
Energy (loss)
Anhedonia (no enjoyment of favourite activities)
Mood state (low, particularly if present on waking)
Feelings of morbid guilt
Feelings of suicidal nature

Care at home

In conjunction with a social worker and the GP you could help to organize:

- nursing care (e.g. district nurse, Macmillan Support Team, Marie Curie nurse, hospice-based day care)
- financial help (e.g. government allowances—disability living allowance, attendance allowance—or grants from charities, e.g. Macmillan Fund, Ex-Serviceman's Fund, etc.)

- practical help (e.g. occupational therapist, home help, meals on wheels, hospital chaplain or local churches, self-help or other voluntary groups).

Hospice care

Hospices provide medical, nursing and spiritual support for the terminally ill and their families. It is important to emphasize that the role of the hospice team is not only to provide support in the terminal stages of cancer, but to initiate and participate in comprehensive symptom control and psychological support. Good symptom control enables some patients referred for 'terminal care' to return to the community, with continuing involvement of the hospice in offering respite care and home visits before perhaps arranging admission to help manage the last few days of life. Avoid using the euphemism 'convalescent home' when you explain to the patient about hospice referral. Try to make time to visit your patient after admission.

ONCOLOGICAL EMERGENCIES

SHOULD YOU RESUSCITATE?

Resuscitation of oncology patients who suffer a cardio-respiratory arrest or become 'shocked' **may not always be appropriate**. This is particularly true when there is no further prospect of effective cancer treatment, or where there is no prospect of a return to an independent enjoyable existence. It is best if these issues are discussed BEFORE THE EVENT. The decision 'not for resuscitation' should always be taken by the **most senior member of the medical team**—it is a decision to be taken **in consultation with the relatives or the patient**—it should be clearly documented and signed in the case notes. It is NOT appropriate for a junior member of the medical or nursing staff to make this decision. If a patient of 'uncertain resuscitation status' collapses—start treatment until senior staff are contacted.

SEPTIC SHOCK

Patients with cancer may be immunosuppressed both because of their tumour and because of chemotherapy-induced neutropenia. It is essential to remember that neutropenic patients may not become pyrexial when septic.

Signs of septic shock	
Non-specifically unwell	Agitation
Pyrexia (*not* inevitable)	Confusion
Hypotension (may appear late)	Altered conscious state
Tachycardia	

Management

Initial
1. High index of suspicion.
2. Establish IV access (preferably central line).
3. Blood and urine cultures (peripheral and central blood).
4. FBC and U&Es.
5. Rapid IV plasma expanders (e.g. Hemacel).
6. Start IV antibiotics (e.g. gentamicin, piperacillin and flucloxacillin or ceftazidime and amikacin).
7. Consider urinary catheterization.
8. Oxygen (**NB**: 24% if COAD or previous bleomycin).

Later
1. Inotropic support if hypotension persists despite adequate plasma expansion.
2. Consider removing Hickman line if suspected infective source and *send tip for culture*.
3. CXR followed by bronchoscopy if appearances suggestive of opportunistic or atypical infection.
4. Blood gas analysis.
5. Physiotherapy if chest infection confirmed.
6. Subcutaneous gCSF if patient is very ill, fails to recover quickly or is beginning a period of prolonged neutropenia.
7. If pyrexia does not settle after 48 h or spikes above 38°C after 48 h, change to second-line antibiotics (e.g. ciprofloxacin and amikacin). Vancomycin should be added if a Gram + infection from an IV line is suspected. *Culture results may be available at this point.*
8. Continue antibiotics until neutrophil count is > 0.5×10^9/L and temperature has been below 37.5° for 48 h.

BLEEDING

Causes
1. Pancytopenia.
2. Clotting diathesis:
   - DIC (especially prostatic cancer)
   - over-anticoagulation
   - abnormal liver function.
3. Acute peptic ulcer.
4. Tumour invasion of major vessel:
   - carotid blow-out with head and neck cancer
   - haemoptysis with lung cancer.

Making the diagnosis
This is usually obvious following history taking and general physical examination. Look particularly for possible causes of pancytopenia or clotting diathesis. In cases of GI haemorrhage, consider urgent oesophago-gastro-duodenoscopy.

Treatment
1. Initial resuscitation:
   - two large-bore IV cannulae
   - cross match
   - check FBC, platelets, clotting screen
   - plasma expanders to maintain BP.

2. Abnormalities of platelets or clotting factors need to be corrected.
3. Major GI haemorrhage—early communication between surgeon, gastroenterologist and oncologist. Early endoscopy. Consider emergency surgery.
4. Major haemoptysis—consider urgent local radiotherapy.
5. Tumour invasion of major vessel, e.g. in head and neck, is a major surgical challenge. Apply pressure to bleeding artery and contact consultant in charge urgently.
6. Appropriateness of resuscitation needs to be considered (see p. 20).

CARDIAC TAMPONADE

Cardiac tamponade is a complication of pericardial effusion and is caused by the restriction of ventricular filling by (usually malignant) fluid of up to 2 L in volume. If the fluid accumulates quickly, a significantly smaller volume may cause symptoms and signs of tamponade.

Common associated tumours
These include breast, lung and lymphoma.

Making the diagnosis
Signs and symptoms • Dyspnoea • Chest pain or 'pressure' • Fatigue • Tachycardia • Low pulse volume • Raised CVP • Cold, sweaty skin ('shut down' appearance) • Pulsus paradoxus—reduction of arterial and pulse pressure on inspiration (> 10 mmHg) • Soft heart sounds • Low urine output.

Investigations • CXR—shows a large globular heart • ECG: sinus tachycardia, low voltage QRS complexes, electrical alternans or 'wandering baseline' • Echocardiogram—demonstrates pericardial fluid and may confirm poor left ventricular contraction.

Treatment
1. If patient is shocked, move to area where there is resuscitative equipment.
2. Raise filling pressure/cardiac output with rapid infusion of normal saline or colloid.
3. Attach ECG monitor.
4. Under ultrasound control, inject local anaesthetic to left of the midline (preferably at 5th or 6th costal interspace) and point needle slightly to the left and cranially to drain a small volume of straw-coloured fluid (**NB**: may be haemorrhagic).
5. Insert larger polythene cannula by the same route and drain up to 500 ml.
6. Send fluid for cytology and culture.

7. Continuous drainage may be necessary if there is more than 500 ml in the pericardial sac—leave plastic venous catheter in situ and connect to an underwater sealed drain with gentle suction applied.

The alternative approach for pericardial drainage is via the xiphisternum, aiming the needle towards the left shoulder. If the pericardial effusion becomes a recurrent problem, the patient should be referred to a cardiothoracic surgeon for creation of a pericardial window to the pleural cavity.

STRIDOR

Stridor is the high-pitched inspiratory (and often expiratory) sound caused by partial laryngeal obstruction. It can be an alarming complication in a patient with carcinoma of the head and neck or a mediastinal tumour involving the trachea.

Differential diagnosis
Acute onset Consider obstructing bolus of food or tumour—perform emergency bronchoscopy.

Breathlessness Look for contributory factors, such as bronchospasm, pulmonary oedema or pleural effusion, and treat.

Management
1. Measure blood gases and/or oxygen saturation. Obtain urgent ENT and anaesthetic opinion. Prepare for urgent bronchoscopy or surgery.
2. Give high-dose dexamethasone to minimize oedema (may be tumour- or treatment-related).

Treatment options
Surgery
- Cricothyroidotomy (e.g. using a percutaneous mini-tracheostomy set)—provides time to make a treatment plan and makes induction of anaesthesia safer.
- Isthmusectomy of the thyroid isthmus in advanced (anaplastic) carcinoma of the thyroid—gives tissue for diagnosis and frees the anterior wall of the trachea from constricting tumour.
- Tracheostomy—consider even for 'incurable' recurrent carcinoma of the head and neck to prevent asphyxia by respiratory obstruction.
- Endoscopic laser vaporization of obstructing tumour—may be useful for obstructing supraglottic tumours to minimize the need for tracheostomy, particularly if given prior to urgent radiotherapy.

Radiotherapy Commence as soon as possible for appropriate tumours, e.g. anaplastic thyroid carcinoma/lymphoma, but bear in mind that stridor may initially be made worse because of reactive oedema.

Chemotherapy Rapid response obtained in small-cell lung carcinoma and lymphoma.

SUPERIOR VENA CAVA OBSTRUCTION

Obstruction of the superior vena cava (SVCO) may be secondary to compression, obstruction or thrombosis of the vessel secondary to a usually malignant process in the superior mediastinum: 70% are due to lung cancers. It may be the presenting feature of a neoplasm. Onset can be rapid, causing considerable distress and fear. The prognosis is dependent upon the underlying diagnosis.

Neoplastic causes
These include carcinoma of the bronchus, lymphoma/leukaemia and germ cell tumours, e.g. testicular teratoma.

Making the diagnosis
Signs and symptoms • Specific: dyspnoea/orthopnoea, swelling of face, neck and upper limbs, venous dilatation over anterior chest wall.
• Associated with underlying condition: cough ± haemoptysis, chest pain, weight loss.

Investigations As the therapeutic approach will be determined by the underlying histological diagnosis, tissue must be obtained for examination in previously undiagnosed patients. This may prove hazardous in a respiratorily compromised patient. Very rarely, immediate treatment is administered on an empirical basis.
   Investigations include:

- CXR—abnormal in > 80% of cases
- biopsy from
    — palpable lymph node, e.g. supraclavicular node *or*
    — bronchoscopy *or*
    — mediastinoscopy *or*
    — thoracotomy
- CT scan of the thorax
- superior vena cavogram—rarely required.

Treatment

Immediate
- Steroids—dexamethasone 16 mg daily.
- Oxygen (**NB**: 24% if background of COAD).

Even gentle sedatives should be used with caution in view of possible respiratory depression.

Specific
Non-small cell lung cancer Median survival is only 2–3 months. Aim to provide immediate adequate palliation of respiratory symptoms with minimum morbidity by external beam radiotherapy. This is usually fractionated, but a single fraction may be adequate.

Chemosensitive tumours Establish histological diagnosis—e.g. lymphoma/ leukaemia, malignant teratoma, small cell lung cancer—and treat underlying condition with appropriate therapy. It may be necessary to modify the first cycle of chemotherapy regimen in a patient who is severely compromised. In most cases there is significant improvement of symptoms within 24–48 h of starting chemotherapy. Subsequent prognosis is determined by histological diagnosis and stage of disease.

Uncertain diagnosis Where histological confirmation of the type of malignancy cannot be obtained, patients should receive an initial short course of external beam radiotherapy. Most patients respond well enough to the radiotherapy to facilitate a histological diagnosis before proceeding to definitive treatment.

Recurrent/non-responsive SVCO SVCO may recur following either radiotherapy or chemotherapy. In patients where there is no scope for more radiotherapy and where the tumour has become resistant to chemotherapy, the prognosis is extremely poor. Occasionally a patient may maintain a good performance status despite recurrent SVCO. In such cases it may be appropriate to consider the insertion of a superior vena caval stent.

Patients with long-term indwelling lines (e.g. Hickman) may develop SVCO secondary to thrombosis. Removal of the line, anticoagulation and occasionally streptokinase or urokinase should resolve the problem. Anticoagulation should continue for 3 months post SVCO.

SPINAL CORD COMPRESSION

Compression of the spinal cord requires rapid assessment and immediate treatment if permanent neurological deficit is to be avoided.

Cancers most commonly giving rise to spinal cord compression • Bronchus • Breast • Prostate • Multiple myeloma • Non-Hodgkin's lymphoma (high grade).

Mechanism of compression
- Extradural compression (most common)
  — e.g. collapse of vertebral body caused by destructive lesion
  — e.g. nodal mass or primary tumour.
- Intradural compression
  — e.g. primary spinal cord tumour
  — e.g. secondary deposit.

Site of spinal cord compression • Thoracic spine—70% • Lumbar spine—20% • Cervical spine—10%.

Making the diagnosis
Signs and symptoms Usually in patients with known metastatic disease, but may occur as the presenting feature of a malignant condition:

- Back pain—may be insidious in onset, but a recent increase in severity should prompt a formal neurological examination. Pain may radiate along the distribution of one or more spinal roots.
- Paraesthesia or sensory loss—below level of compression.
- Bladder symptoms—hesitancy or retention.
- Constipation—may be attributed to opiate analgesics.
- Weakness—the most frightening symptom, usually prompting patient to seek urgent medical help. Lower limbs are more commonly affected, restricting mobility and progressing to complete paralysis within a few days or even hours if left unattended.

Investigations
- Localization of the lesion
  — upper motor neurone deficit below the site of cord compression— usually bilateral
  — impaired sensation below the lesion. **NB**: a lesion at T6 results in a sensory level at T8 with impaired sensation below the T8 dermatome
  — localized tenderness in affected vertebral body.
- Plain X-ray of affected region of spine—may be normal.
- MR scan.
- Myelogram if MR facilities not available.

Tips for physical examination

- Ensure adequate analgesia—a patient in pain will find it difficult to co-operate.
- Test light touch and pin prick descending from normal to abnormal sensation and vice versa in order to obtain reproducible sensory level.
- Always test proprioception—loss of proprioception is prognostic of poor neurological recovery.

Treatment

Following assessment, treatment must be instituted immediately. A delay of several hours may lead to failure of neurological recovery.

1. Dexamethasone 8 mg IV stat.
2. Decide whether surgery or radiotherapy is more appropriate.

Surgery is generally the favoured approach as it offers more rapid decompression, particularly in less radiosensitive tumours (Table 2.1).

TABLE 2.1 Features favouring surgery vs radiotherapy

Surgery	Radiotherapy
Medically fit for surgery	Not fit for surgery
Well-localized site of compression	Multiple sites of compression
Life expectancy > 3 months	Life expectancy < 3 months
Tissue required for diagnosis	Radiosensitive tumour, e.g. lymphoma
Radio-resistant tumour	

Surgery Immediate transfer to neurosurgical unit (patient may require postoperative radiotherapy or chemotherapy depending on diagnosis).

Radiotherapy Emergency treatment required. The possible difficulties encountered in irradiating the patient 'out of hours' are outweighed by the detrimental effect of a few hours' delay. The number of fractions of treatment will depend on the clinical situation.

Outcome

Overall, < 20% of patients achieve a significant neurological improvement. This is primarily due to irreversible neurological damage occurring before initiation of therapy. Realistically, a full recovery can only be expected if the lesion is of < 24 h duration and the neurological loss is not complete at the time of treatment.

CAUDA EQUINA LESIONS

Spinal cord compression may occur anywhere from the foramen magnum to the termination of the cord at L1/L2. Below this level the lumbar and sacral nerve roots form a leash of nerves occupying the spinal canal—the cauda equina. Compression of the cauda equina characteristically presents with root pain followed by lower motor neurone weakness, the distribution of which is dependent on the roots involved. Disturbance of bladder and bowel function is usually late.

RAISED INTRACRANIAL PRESSURE

Raised intracranial pressure (ICP) is usually caused by a space-occupying intracranial lesion, resulting from a secondary deposit or a primary tumour. This may be the presenting episode, or may occur in a patient with a previously diagnosed cancer.

Cerebral metastases are the most frequently occurring intracranial neoplasm.

Common primary sites • Bronchus • Breast • Testicular teratoma • Malignant melanoma • Non-Hodgkin's lymphoma.

Primary intracranial neoplasms • Astrocytomas • Meningiomas • Oligodendrogliomas • Ependymomas • Medulloblastomas • Primary cerebral lymphoma (AIDS-associated) • Pineal tumours • Pituitary tumours.

Clinical features

Symptoms • Headache—characteristically worse on waking • Vomiting—associated with headache, often no significant nausea • Occasionally protracted nausea without vomiting • Visual disturbance • Drowsiness progressing to coma • Convulsions.

Signs • Papilloedema • Raised blood pressure • Bradycardia • Cranial nerve lesions • May be associated with other signs of underlying malignancy, i.e. focal neurological signs due to local pressure effects.

Management

Initial management
1. Reduce cerebral oedema
   • dexamethasone 8 mg IV stat, then 8–12 mg/day
   • consider osmotic diuresis if no response—100–200 ml mannitol 20% infusion 1–2 h.
2. Initiate anticonvulsant treatment where appropriate.

Assessment
CT or MR scan to establish presence, character and number of lesions, then decide on most appropriate intervention.

Specific tumour decompression
Surgery • Complete resection—tumour excision and decompression • Biopsy—for histological confirmation.

Radiotherapy • Curative, i.e. medulloblastoma • Palliative, i.e. metastatic carcinoma. Patients with short life expectancy may benefit from steroids alone.

Chemotherapy Restricted to chemoresponsive tumours, i.e. non-Hodgkin's lymphoma, malignant teratoma and paediatric tumours.

 Patients with cancer can also have benign intracranial lesions, i.e. abscess, when immunosuppressed on cytotoxic therapy.

Outcome
The success of management is dependent on the prognosis of the underlying malignancy.

Curable tumours These include paediatric tumours and low-grade gliomas.

Incurable tumours Where expected survival is only a few months, quality of life may not be improved by radiotherapy. These patients can be managed by steroids alone.

PULMONARY EMBOLUS

The importance of pulmonary embolism (PE) in cancer is related not only to the associated mortality of this treatable condition but also to the fact that dyspnoea is a distressing symptom which may be attributed to other factors in the cancer patient. There may be no sign of a deep venous thrombosis in someone who has multiple PEs.

Causes
• Venous stasis, damage to the vessel wall and alteration in blood coagulability (Virchow's triad).
• In patients with cancer—increased coagulability and stasis (the latter may be secondary to pressure on a vessel either from tumour or from nodes).

Making the diagnosis

Clinical features • Dyspnoea—progressive or sudden • Cough—occasionally with haemoptysis • Chest pain—may be pleuritic or described as a 'weight' • Dizziness—secondary to cardiac arrhythmia/atrial fibrillation (AF) or to postural hypotension • Raised CVP • Wide splitting of the second heart sound • Triple cardiac rhythm—4th heart sound due to forceful atrial contraction because of raised pulmonary pressure. **NB**: not present if there is AF.

Investigations

- ECG—abnormal in 85% of cases and may show any or all of the following
  — S1 Q3 T3 pattern
  — atrial fibrillation
  — partial/complete right bundle branch block.
- CXR—may be normal or may show any of
  — pulmonary atelectasis/wedge-shaped infarcted area
  — 'pruning' of the peripheral pulmonary vessels
  — 'plump' hilar shadow secondary to sharp occlusion of dilated pulmonary artery.
- Arterial blood gases—low PO_2 and low CO_2
  — ventilation/perfusion (VQ) scan will show mismatch in areas of lung ventilation and blood perfusion; may be difficult to interpret if CXR was initially abnormal.
- Pulmonary angiography—the definitive test; only rarely necessary.

Treatment

Points 1–4 pertain mainly to large PEs.

1. Establish IV access and give plasma expanders.
2. Give inhaled oxygen 40% minimum.
3. Inotropes may be needed to improve BP.
4. If large PE compromises the circulation, arrange pulmonary embolectomy or thrombolysis with streptokinase.
5. Anticoagulate with IV heparin. Loading dose usually 5000U; thereafter 1000U/h.
6. Commence oral anticoagulants with warfarin; continue for 3 months.
7. Consider Doppler ultrasound scan to search for lower limb DVT and abdominal ultrasound scan/venogram to look for clot in IVC.

Relative contraindications to anticoagulants	
Patient frailty	Intracranial tumours
Active peptic ulceration	Bladder carcinoma

ACUTE ABDOMEN

The acute abdomen can be caused by inflammation of any intra-abdominal viscus, perforation of a hollow organ, obstruction of the ureter, biliary tract or intestine, rupture of a cyst or tumour, or intestinal infarction. The following are common causes in oncology patients:

- perforation of stomach, duodenum, small bowel, colon (see p. 35).
  NB: steroid therapy may mask inflammatory response and physical signs
- ureteric colic, e.g. tumour lysis, hyperuricaemia
- pancreatitis, e.g. steroid therapy
- urinary retention
- urinary tract infection/cystitis
- basal pneumonia
- tumour infarction or haemorrhage, e.g. hepatoma
- splenic infarction, e.g. CML or NHL
- mesenteric ischaemia, e.g. systemic embolisation or tumour invasion of vessels
- biliary colic.

Rarely, profound neutropenic septicaemia may present as an acute abdomen.

GASTROINTESTINAL OBSTRUCTION

Causes (→ Table 2.2)

TABLE 2.2 Causes of GI obstruction in a patient with cancer	
Large bowel	Primary or recurrent carcinoma of colon or rectum
	Recurrent carcinoma of cervix or ovary
	Pseudo-obstruction (e.g. due to immobility or electrolyte abnormality)
	Anastomotic stricture
	Chronic constipation
Small bowel	Primary lymphoma
	Primary carcinoid
	Secondary malignant melanoma
	Secondary carcinoma of stomach, colon, ovary or breast
	Radiation stricture
	Adhesions

Making the diagnosis

Signs and symptoms

History • Vomiting • Abdominal distension • Colicky abdominal pain
• Constipation.

Examination • Dehydration • Distended abdomen • Visible peristalsis
• Palpable tumour mass • Obstructive bowel sounds • Empty rectum or
palpable mass in rectum or pelvis.

Investigations • FBC • Serum chemistry • Plain AXR • Urgent contrast
enema on unprepared bowel to confirm presence of an obstructing large
bowel lesion.

Treatment

Initial treatment includes: • rehydration, • correction of electrolyte
imbalances, • analgesia and • passage of NG tube.

OBSTRUCTING PRIMARY CARCINOMA

Left colon or rectum

Primary colorectal carcinoma may present with obstruction, precipitating
laparotomy before there has been time to assess, stage or biopsy the tumour.
The surgical strategy if you resect is the same as for elective surgery, i.e. to
include a full lymph node dissection. If unresectable metastatic disease is
present, then node dissection can be omitted.

Treatment options

1. Resection of carcinoma with primary anastomosis—ideal if the surgeon is
   experienced, the patient stable and the peritoneum clean. Optional
   measures to consider, which will reduce the risk of anastomotic leakage:
   • 'on table lavage' of proximal colon to wash out obstructed faeces
   • formation of colostomy or ileostomy proximal to anastomosis
   • extended right hemicolectomy in which entire colon proximal to
     obstruction is resected in order to anastomose terminal ileum to
     descending or sigmoid colon.
2. Resection of carcinoma with anastomosis deferred to a second operation.
   Proximal colon brought to the skin as end-colostomy with distal colon
   either sutured across (rectal stump) or brought to skin (mucus fistula)
   (Hartmann's procedure).
3. Defunctioning colostomy—safe option for a severely ill patient. Transverse
   colon proximal to obstruction is brought out as a loop colostomy, deferring
   resection and anastomosis to a second operation and closure of colostomy
   to a third operation. Also the option for unresectable colorectal tumours
   both primary and secondary.

Right colon or caecum

Treatment options
1. Resection of carcinoma by right hemicolectomy with primary anastomosis—usually possible because of low risk of anastomotic failure.
2. Defunctioning ileostomy—rarely necessary.

OBSTRUCTION IN ADVANCED MALIGNANCY

Large bowel obstruction

Recurrent colorectal, ovarian or cervical carcinoma within the pelvis may cause large bowel obstruction. You will need to decide whether or not there is a realistic chance of salvage therapy being curative in intent as the likelihood of cure is small in patients who have had radical primary treatment with surgery, radiotherapy and/or chemotherapy.

The preoperative workup should include:

- rectal examination
- contrast enema radiology
- CT scan of pelvis and abdomen to give information about the position of the obstructing lesion, resectability and ureter involvement.

Treatment options
1. Resection of the lesion—may involve wider pelvic exenteration if gynaecological or urological organs involved.
2. Proximal 'defunctioning' colostomy leaving the obstruction behind—indicated when disease is irresectable.
3. Conservative treatment—may be chosen by a patient with irresectable disease and short life expectancy, who does not wish the added burden of a colostomy. The aim is to keep the stools as soft as toothpaste. This can be encouraged by high fluid intake, the avoidance of fruit pith and vegetables and the use of a softening laxative such as sodium docusate.

Once the intestinal obstruction has been dealt with, consider risks and benefits of further treatment with radiotherapy or chemotherapy. Dexamethasone and/or octreotide may be of symptomatic benefit to the patient.

SMALL BOWEL OBSTRUCTION

When this occurs in a patient with previous abdominal or pelvic malignancy, conservative treatment with IV fluids and NG aspiration may be attempted for up to 5 days—provided there are no signs of intestinal ischaemia. After this, a laparotomy is usually indicated, particularly as the obstruction may be due to a simple adhesion and not recurrent disease. Preoperative CT scanning is useful to look for extrinsic masses or liver metastases but contrast studies are usually unhelpful.

Treatment options

Resection or by-pass operation • Recurrence—involved loop should be resected (ideal) or bypassed with side-to-side anastomosis • Multiple sites of obstruction—if all sites are bypassed, patient may develop diarrhoea, malabsorption or blind loop syndrome; but if an obstructing site is missed, operation will not work or, worse, will result in an anastomotic leak and fistula.

Defunctioning ileostomy as alternative to bypass Created proximal to first obstructed loop where multiple loop obstruction. Not every patient with terminal disease will wish this option.

Non-operative option • Analgesia • Antiemetics • NG tube optional depending upon symptoms • Dexamethasone ± octreotide may be of symptomatic benefit to the patient.

GASTRIC OUTLET OBSTRUCTION

This is seen in conditions such as carcinoma of the pancreas or distal stomach.

Treatment options
Resection if possible

Gastroenterostomy May be performed laparoscopically. Once obstruction has been resolved, consider other treatment modalities, e.g. chemotherapy with carcinoma of stomach.

Conservative treatment Look for electrolyte abnormalities due to loss of H^+, K^+ and CL^-. Dexamethasone and motility agents have little to offer, but an antiemetic may reduce nausea.

RADIATION-INDUCED STRICTURE

This typically arises because of small bowel damage caused by pelvic irradiation (especially intracavitary for carcinoma of the cervix) 1–5 years after treatment. If surgery is necessary, then care should be taken to avoid an anastomosis that includes a loop of bowel damaged by the radiation field.

GASTROINTESTINAL PERFORATION

Making the diagnosis

Signs and symptoms
History • Sudden onset of abdominal pain, usually constant and severe.

Examination • Tachycardia • Hypotension • Rebound tenderness
• Rigid abdomen • Absent bowel sounds.

Investigations
CXR (erect)—the absence of subdiaphragmatic air does not exclude
perforation and a diagnosis may be made on clinical features alone.

Treatment
Urgent laparotomy is the wisest option unless the patient is known to be in
the terminal stages of disease or is myelosuppressed following chemotherapy.
The patient could have a benign condition such as a perforated peptic ulcer.
Patients with intestinal lymphoma who respond rapidly to chemotherapy are
at risk of perforation. Steroids—part of most lymphoma regimens—may
mask the usual clinical signs. If progressive signs of peritonitis develop then
laparotomy is advisable.

Perforation as a presenting symptom of gastric or colonic carcinoma is
associated with locally advanced disease and a poor prognosis. If the patient
is stable, complete surgical clearance should be attempted as with elective
surgery for these conditions.

HYPERCALCAEMIA

Tumour-associated hypercalcaemia is due to an imbalance between bone
resorption and calcium excretion. A rapid rise in serum calcium is more likely
to result in symptoms, which are rare if the serum level is < 3.2 mmol/L.
A high index of suspicion is required to diagnose hypercalcaemia because it
may be relatively 'silent' until very severe.

Symptoms
Check serum calcium if any of the following are present: • thirst • polyuria
• anorexia • nausea • headache • constipation • mental blunting/
confusion • cardiac dysrhythmia.

Tumours most commonly associated with hypercalcaemia: • breast
• myeloma • renal • non-small cell lung cancer • lymphoma • prostate.

Causes
These include: • bone metastases • PTH-related peptide secretion by
the tumour • dehydration • drugs (e.g. thiazide diuretics, hormonal
treatments in breast cancer—including tamoxifen) • immobilization.

Treatment
This is not related to the cause of the hypercalcaemia.

1. IV hydration with 1 L normal saline 4-hourly and adequate K^+ for at least
   24 h, then 1 L bag of normal saline or dextrose 6-hourly for a further 48–72 h.
2. Check for signs of left ventricular failure at least twice daily during
   hyperhydration, give frusemide 20–40 mg IV if necessary.
3. Weigh patient daily if possible.
4. Watch for fall in serum albumin which will cause ankle oedema and may
   be mistaken for fluid overload.
5. If calcium is still high at 24 h give bisphosphonate (e.g. pamidronate
   30–60 mg).

 Some centres give bisphosphonates before the 24 h timepoint, but
adequate hydration is always essential.

6. Alternative drugs are
   • prednisolone 60 mg daily: of questionable effectiveness and can cause
     tumour lysis
   • salmon calcitonin 200 IU 8-hourly: expensive and transiently effective
   • mithramycin 25 µg/kg IV × 3 weekly—delayed effect and results in
     thrombocytopenia and renal toxicity.

When hypercalcaemia has been resolved, commence appropriate treatment
of the underlying tumour as soon as possible. If hypercalcaemia is diagnosed
in a patient with a relapsed untreatable tumour it may not be appropriate to
correct it.

The prognosis of patients with tumour-related hypercalcaemia is generally
poor with, in breast cancer patients, a median survival of 8 months.

PATHOLOGICAL FRACTURES

Sustained through a bone weakened by malignant infiltration from a primary tumour or a metastatic deposit (may occasionally be presenting symptom) (Table 2.3).

TABLE 2.3 Causes of pathological fracture

Metastatic disease	Bone tumour
Breast	Multiple myeloma
Prostate	Osteosarcoma
Lung	Ewing's sarcoma
Thyroid	Lymphoma
Kidney	Chondrosarcoma

Making the diagnosis
Signs and symptoms • Pain—sudden onset often associated with minimal trauma, or may appear spontaneously affecting long bones or axial skeleton • Displacement and loss of function of the affected limb • Collapsed vertebral body may give rise to spinal cord compression (see pp. 26–28).

Treatment
1. Analgesia.
2. X-ray to confirm diagnosis.
3. Surgery
   — biopsy for histological diagnosis
   — internal fixation, e.g. shaft of femur/humerus
   — joint replacement occasionally appropriate, e.g. femoral/humoral head.

Prevention
Pathological fracture often occurs in patients with known metastatic disease, and prophylactic measures may be taken in patients at risk.

Lytic lesion in long bone Monitor response to systemic or radiation treatment radiologically.

Progression of lytic process Consider prophylactic pinning or plating of lesion.

OSTEORADIONECROSIS

This condition starts as an aseptic necrosis caused by radiotherapy damage, but it may progress to secondary infection with ulceration, cellulitis and discharging sinuses or fistulae. Risk increased by trauma to bone previously treated with high-dose radiation—e.g. tooth extraction leading to osteoradionecrosis of the mandible. Internal fixation should be considered, but once secondary infection has developed then resection of the bone and perhaps amputation may become inevitable.

ACUTE CONFUSIONAL STATES

The essential feature of an acute confusional state which differentiates it from an acute anxiety state, a psychotic episode or a chronic brain syndrome (e.g. dementia), is *impairment of consciousness*. The confusional state characteristically has an abrupt onset, with disorientation in time and place and occasionally also in person which often fluctuates in intensity. The clinical course is usually short-lived once the cause has been treated, and there is often complete amnesia for the events that took place while confused. Hallucinations, visual illusions and persecutory delusions are common, the delusions usually being directed against close relatives or attending medical and nursing staff. Response to questioning is slow, and the patient is unable to sustain a logical sentence.

Do not regard an acute confusional state as a diagnosis in itself, but rather as a *symptom* of some underlying and potentially treatable organic problem.

Important causes
- Metabolic
  - — hypercalcaemia (e.g. breast, myeloma)
  - — acute renal failure (e.g. cervix, prostate, bladder)
  - — hypoglycaemia or hyperglycaemia (e.g. steroid therapy)
  - — hyponatraemia (e.g. small cell lung carcinoma).
- Sepsis
  - — septicaemia (e.g. neutropenic patient)
  - — unrecognized abscess (e.g. lung, brain, intra-abdominal).
- Hypoxia.
- Chest infection.
- PE.
- 'Silent' MI.

- Drugs
  - alcohol withdrawal
  - tranquillizers and sedatives
  - drug combinations.
- Brain metastases.

Management

Rushing in with physical restraint and a hefty dose of IM sedation should be avoided: such a confrontation might simply convince the patient that his paranoid delusions are correct! Gentle reassurance is often effective, reserving pharmacological sedation for those whose behaviour disrupts investigations or therapy. Many confused patients actually become withdrawn rather than aggressive.

Investigations

- Screen for metabolic disturbance, sepsis and hypoxia—all potent causes of confusion.
- The 'delirium tremens' of acute alcohol withdrawal is recognizable from the history, from a raised mean cell volume and from the characteristic tremor.
- Night sedation in the elderly, particularly the combination of a benzodiazepine with an opiate, is a potent cause of a confusional state.

Once you have excluded these, arrange a brain scan to look for metastases.

Acute confusional state: plan of management

Look for the cause
- History
- Examination
- Investigations
  - metabolic: FBC, U&E, sugar, calcium
  - sepsis: FBC, blood culture, CXR
  - hypoxia: blood gases, ECG
  - brain metastases: CT scan, lumbar puncture if raised ICP excluded
- Once you have found the likely cause, treat vigorously.

Reassure
- Place the patient in a well-lit side room, do not leave unattended.
- Encourage relatives to sit with the patient.
- Maintain day/night routine with familiar staff and relatives.

Sedate
Appropriate sedative drugs include:
- promazine 25–200 mg orally and repeat 8-hourly; *or*
- haloperidol 5 mg IM, repeated hourly if necessary, *or*
- chlormethiazole, perphenazine, chlorpromazine.

Avoid benzodiazepines and sedative drug combinations.

HYPERKALAEMIA

Aetiology

Acute renal failure due to:

- bilateral ureteric obstruction (the commonest cause in oncology patients—see below)
- septicaemia (pp. 20–21)
- tumour lysis syndrome
- graft versus host disease (pp. 41–42).

Factors that need to be excluded:

- drug therapy (e.g. potassium-sparing diuretics, ACE-inhibitors, potassium supplements)
- adrenal insufficiency (e.g. due to bilateral adrenal metastases)
- haemolyzed blood sample ('pseudohyperkalaemia').

Treatment

Emergency

Plasma K^+ of > 7 mmol/L is a medical emergency. An ECG should be performed to look for (in order of severity):

1. tenting of T waves
2. loss of P waves
3. widening of QRS
4. slurring of ST segment
5. sine wave pattern that precedes cardiac arrest.

If ECG abnormalities present, immediate management includes:

- 10 ml 10% calcium gluconate given over 2 min (may be repeated up to 30 ml)
- IV glucose (50 g) and insulin 15 units soluble bolus infusions
- 100 ml 4.2% sodium bicarbonate.

If normal ECG, calcium gluconate can be omitted. The above measures will control hyperkalaemia for 2–3 h.

Maintenance

- Calcium resonium enemas 20 g 8-hourly.
- Dialysis.
- treat underlying cause where appropriate.

URETERIC OBSTRUCTION

Causes
These include:

- primary carcinoma of ureter, bladder or prostate
- invasion of ureter by advanced pelvic tumour, e.g. carcinoma of cervix
- ureteric calculus.

Making the diagnosis
Ureteric obstruction may cause loin pain or secondary pyelonephritis, but often the onset is insidious and painless. Bilateral obstruction may present with symptoms of renal failure. The diagnosis can be confirmed by renal ultrasound, and a plain abdominal X-ray should be performed to exclude a calculus.

Treatment
Unilateral obstruction by an extrinsic tumour usually requires a bypass procedure using a 'double J' stent in order to prevent renal infection or parenchymal damage. Bilateral ureteric obstruction or obstruction of a solitary kidney is a surgical emergency requiring close collaboration with a urologist and interventional radiologist. Once the haemoglobin, serum K^+ and clotting studies are normalised the plan of treatment will be as follows:

1. Locate level of obstruction by ultrasound or CT scan.
2. Perform cystoscopy under GA and confirm diagnosis by ureteroscopy or retrograde pyelography.
3. Insert ureteric 'double J' stent across stenosis.
4. If stent insertion unsuccessful, or patient unfit for GA, perform percutaneous nephrostomy—one side is usually sufficient—on the kidney with the most cortex.

Intervention may not be appropriate, e.g. in untreatable relapse of advanced carcinoma of cervix. This dilemma should be discussed frankly with the patient and relatives.

GRAFT VERSUS HOST DISEASE

Acute graft versus host disease (GVHD) is one of the major complications of allogeneic bone marrow transplantations, occurring in up to 50% of ALL patients and with a mortality rate of around 25%. It is defined as the reaction of the donor graft T lymphocytes—CD4+, DC8+ and natural killer (NK) cells—against the host non-major HLA antigens.

- A mild degree of GVH reaction is favoured because there is also a graft vs leukaemia effect which reduces the risk of tumour relapse.
- Autologous GVHD can occur spontaneously or following low-dose cyclosporin.

Grading
I   Skin erythema
II   Skin blistering
III–IV   Multiple organ involvement

Making the diagnosis
Signs and symptoms • Acute erythema of palms, soles, face ± scrotum.

Treatment
Initial treatment methylprednisolone 1 g/day × 3 d, to be reviewed and reduced gradually as erythema resolves.

Prophylaxis • Methotrexate days 1–100 post transplant • Cyclosporin ± methotrexate until day 11 post transplant • Remove mediating T cells by purging bone marrow grafts (initially through use of monoclonal antibody Campath-1G) • High-dose pentoxifylline to reduce secretion of cytokines TNF (which mediate the activation of effector cells) • Monoclonal anti-TNF-alpha antibody in severe acute GVHD—no complete responses have been seen and the condition recurs on cessation of treatment.

CHRONIC GVHD
Longer term, a failure of discrimination between self and non-self occurs in approximately 30% of transplant recipients. This can lead to intractable diarrhoea, deranged liver function, impaired renal function and CNS symptoms.

Treatment
- Steroids can be helpful.
- Thalidomide was found to be well tolerated and effective in early studies and is currently under further evaluation.

PROBLEMS IN PRACTICE

ALOPECIA

Hair loss is caused by a number of chemotherapy agents (Table 3.1) and by cranial irradiation. It results from a direct cytotoxic effect on dividing cells within hair follicles, and usually commences 2 weeks after treatment has been started. The drugs most likely to cause temporary alopecia are alkylating agents, antibiotic antimitotics, nitrosoureas and taxanes.

Patients should be warned if the drugs being administered cause alopecia, and arrangements made at the earliest possible opportunity to supply a wig for the period of alopecia. Hair regrowth starts around 2 months after completion of chemotherapy.

Scalp cooling may prevent or retard expected hair loss when drugs have a short half-life (e.g. doxorubicin) but it is not recommended where there may be meningeal involvement (e.g. leukaemia). It produces vasoconstriction of the scalp veins before and shortly after the period of peak plasma drug concentration. Reducing scalp temperature to 23°C, commencing 10 min before the drug is given and continuing 30 min afterwards, will usually prevent hair loss. Scalp cooling does not prevent alopecia in patients who have abnormal liver function, for example secondary to liver metastases.

TABLE 3.1 Drugs commonly causing alopecia

Alopecia inevitable	• Doxorubicin
	• Epirubicin
	• Etoposide
	• Ifosfamide
Alopecia possible	• Cyclophosphamide (e.g. CMF)

ASCITES

The commonest causes of malignant ascites are carcinoma of the ovary and carcinomas of the gastrointestinal tract, but any tumour which metastasizes into the peritoneal cavity, liver or omentum may present with this complication.

Ascites in an oncology patient is usually due to intraperitoneal tumour, but other causes to be considered are tuberculous peritonitis, constrictive pericarditis, cirrhosis of the liver and Budd–Chiari syndrome.

Making the diagnosis

Signs and symptoms • Increasing abdominal girth and distension
• Weight gain • Bilateral ankle oedema • Shifting dullness and fluid thrill.

Investigations • Abdominal ultrasound to confirm the presence of ascites;
often demonstrates the site of primary or secondary tumour • Diagnostic
paracentesis ('ascitic tap') should be performed and fluid sent for cytological
examination as well as bacteriology.

Treatment

The treatment of malignant ascites involves a stepwise progression.

1. Treat underlying condition (e.g. commence chemotherapy for ovarian
   carcinoma).
2. Begin diuretic therapy. Some patients with malignant ascites will respond to
   this measure. Commence with a small dose of spironolactone (e.g. 100 mg
   daily) and monitor response by regular weighing of the patient, aiming
   for weight loss of 0.5 kg/day. If no response is achieved, then increase
   spironolactone to 100 mg 12-hourly and then 100 mg 8-hourly. As a final
   measure introduce frusemide at 20 mg daily rising to 120 mg daily. In
   patients receiving frusemide, ensure adequate fluid intake and monitor
   serum creatinine and Na.
3. Perform therapeutic paracentesis. If diuretic therapy fails, or
   decompression of ascites is required for symptomatic relief of respiratory
   embarrassment, then a therapeutic ascitic tap may be performed. The
   abdomen should be cleansed with antiseptic, and using a full sterile
   technique a fine cannula (e.g. peritoneal dialysis catheter) is introduced
   into the peritoneal cavity. The site of the ascitic tap should be within an
   area of dullness on percussion, perhaps under ultrasound control, avoiding
   the surface marking of the inferior epigastric artery. Introduce the trochar
   and catheter gradually through the abdominal wall with gentle aspiration,
   until straw-coloured fluid is drawn back. A drainage bag is attached and
   the ascites slowly decompressed. Following this procedure, it is important
   to monitor the patient's pulse and blood pressure since there may be a fall
   in the intravascular volume; in the elderly it may be wise to have an IV
   infusion in situ.
4. Insert a peritoneal–venous shunt. For refractory cases requiring regular
   therapeutic paracentesis, a shunt between the peritoneal cavity and the
   venous system may be inserted surgically. Subclinical DIC may occur.
   Fluid overload is avoided by draining ascites at time of shunt insertion.

Complications of paracentesis

- Catheter falls out (inadequately secured!)
- Catheter-related sepsis with peritonitis
  — culture fluid and catheter, commence IV antibiotics
- Loculation (after repeated paracentesis)
- Seeding of tumour (onto abdominal wall)
- Perforation of viscus (abdominal pain, signs of sepsis, silent abdomen)
  — if suspected, remove the peritoneal catheter and commence IV antibiotics; watch carefully for signs of increasing peritonitis
  — consider laparotomy
- Hypoalbuminaemia

Chemotherapy and ascites
Exercise caution in administering IV chemotherapy to patients with ascites since the drugs may accumulate in the ascitic fluid. In the case of methotrexate this 'third space phenomenon' can increase toxicity markedly.

Intraperitoneal chemotherapy (e.g. cisplatin) has been used to treat malignant ascites, but few patients gain long-term benefit. If intraperitoneal cisplatin is to be used, renal function must be monitored.

CARCINOID SYNDROME

Carcinoid tumours arise from the enterochromaffin cells which are scattered mainly throughout the intestine and main bronchi. Peptides synthesized by carcinoid tumours include 5-hydroxytryptamine (5-HT), 5-hydroxytryptophan and ACTH. Secretions vary with the site of the carcinoid, and those situated in the foregut (including bronchi) are most frequently associated with the symptoms known as the carcinoid syndrome. The carcinoid syndrome is a manifestation of advanced disease.

Making the diagnosis
Signs and symptoms • Palpable abdominal mass or hepatomegaly (66% of patients) • Cutaneous flushing (95%, duration from min to hours) • Diarrhoea (85%) • Asthma or wheezing (25%) • Valvular heart disease secondary to endocardial fibrosis (50%) • Facial telangiectasia • Intestinal obstruction or rectal bleeding • Occasionally, hepatic capsular pain from gross hepatomegaly, usually with normal liver function tests.

Investigations • Carcinoid tumours may be an incidental finding in histological examination of a resected appendix • Urinary concentrations of 5-hydroxyindoleacetic acid (5-HIAA, a major metabolite of 5-HT)

> 8 mg/24 hours (sensitive measurement in 75% of cases) are elevated. Levels are directly related to tumour volume ● 5-HT levels can also be measured in plasma and urine.

Treatment

Symptom relief ● 5-HT antagonists ● Standard antidiarrhoeals (e.g. loperamide) ● Continuous infusion somatostatin or subcutaneous injection of synthetic derivative is helpful in around 90% of patients.

Surgery Resect tumour wherever possible.

Chemotherapy Unresectable disease (e.g. multiple liver metastases):
● Single-agent chemotherapy with 5-fluorouracil, doxorubicin, cyclophosphamide or streptozotocin—tumour response approximately 25%. There is no proven benefit in combination therapy.
● Interferon has documented response rate of ≤40%.

Prognosis

Survival rates depend on the site and extent of the tumour, up to 80% at 5 years:

● median survival from onset of symptoms 3.5–8 years
● patients may survive 30 years from time of diagnosis.

    The level of 5-HIAA correlates with survival.

CARDIOMYOPATHY

Cardiomyopathy may result from chemotherapy—the drugs implicated are the anthracyclines, e.g. doxorubicin—or radiotherapy. The mechanism of cardiac damage is through free radical generation, and symptomatic cardiomyopathy is rarely seen at cumulative doses < 450 mg/m², although at cumulative doses of 700 mg/m², the incidence rises to 40%.

Risk factors
● High-dose cyclophosphamide—may induce a cardiac toxicity independent of cardiomyopathy resulting from anthracycline delivery.
● Concurrent or prior mediastinal irradiation (many years previously).

Making the diagnosis
Signs and symptoms Cardiomyopathy is manifested typically 30–60 d after the last dose of anthracycline, but may occur years after treatment with doxorubicin. Features include:

- Congestive cardiac failure—most common manifestation of the disease.
- Histological changes—initially a focal area of degenerated cells, may be replaced by fibrosis.
- Changes are seen in almost all patients receiving cumulative doses of 240 mg/m^2 doxorubicin.

Investigations MUGA radionucleotide scan before and during anthracycline treatment to assess LVEF in elderly patients or in those with a cardiac history (normal 50% with > 5% on exercising). Repeat in higher-risk patients receiving anthracycline after every 100 mg/m^2 dose delivered.

Preventive measures
- Limit cumulative dose delivered (see above).
- Use one of the newer anthracyclines, e.g. epirubicin.
- Give cardioprotectant to higher-risk patients to reduce free radical generation.

CONSTIPATION

Constipation is a common symptom in cancer patients through any or all of the following mechanisms: • drugs, e.g. opiate analgesics, vinca alkaloids • immobility • bowel obstruction • cord compression • hypercalcaemia • dehydration, possibly secondary to nausea or vomiting • diet low in fibre.

Making the diagnosis
May present as faecal incontinence or overflow diarrhoea.

Taking the history
Include specific questions about: • the patient's normal bowel habit • duration of constipation • diet • mobility • drug history • vomiting (proximal obstruction) • absolute constipation (distal obstruction).

 Symptoms associated with hypercalcaemia may be absent where onset is gradual.

Examination and investigation • Digital rectal examination • Plain AXR to confirm constipation • Fluid levels on erect X-ray or dilated small bowel loops indicate intestinal obstruction rather than constipation.

Management
Depends on aetiology.

Mild cases
- Encourage increased mobility and fluid intake.
- Prescribe bulking agents (e.g. Fybogel or co-danthrusate 4 tabs 12-hourly or suspension).

With opiate analgesics
Oral and rectal medication are required in most cases. These include:

- Prophylactic laxatives
  — explain the reason for taking them
  — Normax: warn about red urine discoloration
  — Lactulose: usually prescribed as second line after Normax, an osmotically active agent requiring regular ingestion.
- Magnesium sulphate 10 ml orally 6-hourly and rectally if no result in 48 h—usually resolves in 4 h.
- Glycerol/bisacodyl suppositories and phosphate enemas if distal faecal mass.

Constipation due to chemotherapy
Usually resolves spontaneously within 10 days.

Mechanical obstruction
- Stop all stimulant laxatives to avoid exacerbation of abdominal pain (not always present).
- The following may be necessary:
  — nasogastric suction
  — IV fluids
  — surgical opinion
  — barium enema—may reveal occlusion by tumour necessitating surgical intervention.
- Conservative management—may be appropriate in patients with known peritoneal disease and advanced, incurable cancer (e.g. previously treated ovarian carcinoma).
- Steroids to reduce oedema associated with obstruction.

DIARRHOEA

Causes
These include: • chemotherapy-induced • infective diarrhoea • pseudomembranous colitis • radiation enteritis or proctitis • GI fistula, e.g. gastro-colic • overflow diarrhoea secondary to faecal impaction, e.g. opiates.

Making the diagnosis
1. Abdominal and rectal examination.
2. Microscopy and culture of stool.
3. Sigmoidoscopy.
4. Plain abdominal X-ray.
5. *Clostridium difficile* serology.

Treatment
- Maintain hydration and electrolyte balance.
- Treat the cause.
- Anti-diarrhoeal medication if necessary but try to avoid.

HAEMORRHAGIC CYSTITIS

Radiation or chemotherapy may induce dysuria and micro-or macroscopic haematuria.

CHEMOTHERAPY-INDUCED MECHANISMS

Both cyclophosphamide and ifosfamide may cause haemorrhagic cystitis. Cyclophosphamide is a cytotoxic alkylating agent which is metabolized into chlorethylazairidine and acrolein. The metabolites, which are activated by the liver and excreted into the urine, react with the bladder endothelium during storage in the bladder prior to voiding.

Making the diagnosis
Signs and symptoms Symptoms may develop months after therapy has been completed, and incidence may be higher with chronic oral administration than with intermittent IV use. Look for: • mucosal oedema • haemorrhage • ulceration • bladder fibrosis • acute haemorrhagic cystitis—induced by high-dose cyclophosphamide ($\leq 12\%$).

Prevention
- Adequate hydration while cyclophosphamide is being delivered.
- Diuresis maintained with diuretics as drug may cause direct tubular toxicity.
- For patients receiving ifosfamide or high-dose cyclophosphamide, daily IV administration of MESNA (sodium 2-mercaptoethanesulphonate), both before and during therapy, at 160% of the total dose of cyclophosphamide delivered (prevents formation of acrolein and binds to any acrolein present).

RADIATION-INDUCED

Can occur when high doses of radiation are administered to the pelvis.
Severity is dependent on the dose and volume of bladder irradiated.
Symptoms usually resolve within 3–4 weeks following completion of therapy.
A reduction in bladder capacity can occur many months following treatment
due to fibrotic changes in the bladder wall.

INFERTILITY AND CONTRACEPTION

The young age of some patients with cancer means that the effect of treatment
on future fertility must be considered. This is especially important where
treatment may be curative, e.g. leukaemia, Hodgkin's lymphoma. The drugs
most likely to result in infertility are the alkylating agents.

Male patients

Points to consider:

- Spermatogenesis reduced by chemotherapy without effect on the Leydig
  and Sertoli cells.
- Potency maintained, although those with advanced teratoma, leukaemia or
  lymphoma may have reduced sperm counts.
- Sperm banking should be offered to all male patients before chemotherapy
  or gonadal irradiation.
- Men should be advised to delay fathering children for at least 3 months
  because of possible teratogenic effects.

Female patients

Points to consider:

- Menstrual periods can become irregular or cease during chemotherapy.
- In women > 40 years periods are likely to cease permanently.
- In younger women periods may return up to 2 years after completion
  of treatment.
- Despite menstrual irregularity or amenorrhoea, women of child-bearing
  age should take contraceptive precautions during treatment.
- Women may have normal pregnancies after completion of chemotherapy,
  without increased risk of teratogenesis.
- All women who have pelvic irradiation are rendered permanently infertile.

Children
Points to consider:

- Chemotherapy given before puberty rarely causes infertility.
- Gonadal irradiation inevitably renders the child infertile.

MUCOSITIS

Risk factors
- Chemotherapy-induced neutropenia—encourages candidiasis.
- Drug-induced mucosal sloughing—causes pain and dysphagia.
- Neutropenia in association with dental or gingival infection—increases the risk of systemic sepsis.
- Radiotherapy—reduces salivary secretions, causing dry mouth, debris collection and infection risk.

Prevention
Good oral hygiene is imperative in cancer patients. All patients receiving high-dose chemotherapy, 5-fluorouracil infusion, radiotherapy or surgery to the oral cavity or salivary glands should see a dental hygienist before treatment commences.

Mucositis is best prevented by:

- regular tooth-brushing (NB: soft brush if platelets are low)
- chlorhexidine gluconate (Corsodyl) mouthwash 6-hourly
- artificial saliva if the mouth is dry
- prophylactic nystatin suspension
- amphotericin lozenges.

Treatment
- Stop 5-FU infusion (where appropriate).
- Continue regular mouth care.
- Prescribe Acyclovir for ulcers suggestive of herpes simplex.
- Diamorphine by subcutaneous infusion for severe pain.
- Oral fluconazole for oral candidiasis.
- Sucralfate suspension for painful mucositis (obviates need for H2-antagonists).
- Continue treatment until symptoms have resolved—either naturally if post 5-FU or radiotherapy or on recovery of WBC count post high-dose chemotherapy.

NAUSEA AND VOMITING

Causes (→ Table 3.2)

TABLE 3.2 Nausea and vomiting: causes	
Biochemical	Uraemia
	Hypercalcaemia
	Hyponatraemia
Mechanical	Intestinal obstruction
	Gastric outlet obstruction
	Peptic ulceration
Neurological	Raised ICP
	Brain metastases
Treatment-related	Analgesia, e.g. opiates
	Cytotoxic drugs
	Abdominal irradiation

Making the diagnosis
Management depends on the aetiology, which must be ascertained by history, including an accurate drug history, full clinical examination and relevant investigations.

Investigations • Blood chemistry—to exclude hypercalcaemia, hyponatraemia and uraemia • AXR—to exclude intestinal obstruction • Endoscopy—to exclude peptic ulceration • CT brain scan—to exclude brain metastases • CT scan of abdomen and pelvis—in patients with ovarian cancer may reveal diffuse peritoneal involvement and high risk of subacute intestinal obstruction.

Treatment
- Mechanical obstruction
  - — NG tube
  - — IV fluids
  - — assess requirement for surgical intervention.
- Biochemical imbalance, brain metastases, peptic ulceration—correct as standard practice.
- Pharmacology
  - — if patient is taking opiates, reassess and alter dosage as necessary
  - — prescribe regular simple antiemetics, e.g. metoclopramide, for regular or intermittent use.

CHEMOTHERAPY-INDUCED NAUSEA

Cytotoxic treatment is notorious for causing nausea and vomiting and is one of the patient's greatest fears associated with this treatment modality. The emetogenicity of drugs varies, with cisplatin one of the most emetic drugs (90% of patients within 6 h of administration).

An improved understanding of the physiology of vomiting has facilitated development of more effective antiemetics.

Types of emesis

Acute Immediately following therapy with duration up to 24 h. The mechanism is through receptors in the gut wall which, through visceral innervation, particularly the vagus nerve, stimulate the centrally situated nucleus tractus solitarious or 'vomiting centre' in the caudal part of the fourth ventricle.

Delayed This peaks at 48–72 h after cisplatin and may last for 1 week or longer. The mechanism is not well understood.

Anticipatory There are multiple causes of anticipatory vomiting. Even the thought of chemotherapy or the sight or smell of the hospital where chemotherapy has been given may induce vomiting. The best management of anticipatory vomiting is its prevention through adequate management/prevention of emesis on the first cycle of chemotherapy.

Treatment

- Pretreatment with antiemetics before delivery of chemotherapy is essential.
- The recommended antiemetics depend on the emetogenicity of the drug combination.
- For regimens of low emetogenicity, standard drugs like metoclopramide and dexamethasone will be effective:
  — IV administration pre- or during treatment
  — oral preparations for 3 d following chemotherapy.
- Anxious patients may benefit from the antiemetic and relaxant effect of a single dose of lorazepam pre-chemotherapy.
- Haloperidol and chlorpromazine are more rarely used but are effective antiemetics in high-dose therapy or intractable nausea and vomiting.

5-HT$_3$ receptor antagonists

These antiemetics—ondansetron, granisetron and tropisetron—all act through blocking the release of 5-hydroxytryptamine (5-HT) from the enterochromaffin cells from the mucosa of the upper GI tract.

- Recommended for first-line use in patients who are to receive highly emetic chemotherapy, e.g. cisplatin, cyclophosphamide and dacarbazine.
- Oral and IV administration equally effective.
- Addition of steroids (dexamethasone) increases efficacy.

NEUROPATHY

Peripheral neuropathy may be a paraneoplastic condition but is also a complication seen with several anticancer drugs. The main agents are vincristine, vindesine and, more rarely, cisplatin, vinblastine, procarbazine and taxol. Elderly patients are especially susceptible to the cumulative neurotoxicity of the vinca alkaloids. Peripheral neuropathy is often irreversible and can be very disabling.

Making the diagnosis
Signs and symptoms • Loss of the deep tendon reflexes—earliest sign (**NB**: their frequent absence in elderly patients can be misleading) • May present as a burning in the fingers or the toes • Less commonly, the patient complains of difficulty in doing up buttons—suggests a more advanced problem • Foot drop in extreme cases.

Management
- Substitute vinblastine for vincristine.
- Discontinue cisplatin and taxol.

Vincristine also causes autonomic neuropathy. The dose should be reduced, omitted or substituted if intestinal obstruction ('vincristine gut') presents following chemotherapy.

NEUTROPENIA

Neutropenia is strictly defined as a polymorphonuclear neutrophil count of $< 0.5 \times 10^9/L$. The blood count is at its nadir 10–14 d following treatment with chemotherapy.

> ⚠ Prior to commencing each course of chemotherapy, FBC must be checked. Patients and relatives must be warned of the possibility of neutropenia with the attendant risks of infection. If the WBC count is low there may not be a pyrexia.

Making the diagnosis
Any patient on chemotherapy who complains of • fever • rigor • fatigue • dizziness • confusion • agitation • malaise—should be seen immediately for a FBC and examination.

Management
As for septic shock (see pp. 20–21).

NUTRITION

Weight loss is common due to anorexia, dysphagia or as a systemic manifestation of disease. Cancer treatments are often arduous, tending to reduce dietary intake further, and for these reasons nutritional support is important.

Enteral feeding
Able to swallow? Give high-calorie, high-protein dietary supplements.

Unable to swallow? Consider:
1. analgesia before meals
2. relief of dysphagia by endoscopically placed stent, laser therapy, etc.
3. fine-bore NG tube
4. gastrostomy (ideally by PEG)
5. jejunostomy.

Prescribe commercially available enteral solution in collaboration with the dietician. Start with a dilute solution to avoid precipitating diarrhoea. Weigh the patient weekly.

Parenteral feeding
This may be necessary for patients in whom the GI tract is unsuitable for feeding. Parenteral feeding solutions should be prescribed in liaison with the dietician and pharmacy.

- Best undertaken using a tunnelled central line.
- Monitor weight twice weekly.
- Monitor biochemistry twice weekly including calcium, phosphate.
- Monitor blood sugar daily.
- Monitor zinc and magnesium levels as necessary.

Is nutritional support always appropriate?
Nutritional intervention is an appropriate form of 'life support' where the underlying disease state is potentially reversible. It is difficult to justify a feeding gastrostomy in a patient with advancing and incurable carcinoma of the oesophagus.

Cancer diet?
Patients often ask if any dietary measures can improve their outcome, and there has been media interest in diets promoted by alternative/complementary

practitioners. The consensus view is that a balanced diet including vitamin supplements in moderation is worthwhile, but more extreme 'cancer diets' are not recommended.

OPPORTUNISTIC INFECTIONS

When a patient is immunosuppressed through tumour or treatment for a protracted period of time (> 21 d), the risk of opportunistic infection increases significantly (Table 3.3). This is a major problem in allogeneic bone marrow transplants where prolonged immunosuppressive therapy (cyclosporin, steroid, etc.) is required to prevent marrow rejection. The recommended practice to reduce the risk of one of the commonest opportunistic infections, *Pneumocystis pneumoniae*, is to prescribe co-trimoxazole 1 tablet 12-hourly 3 times weekly. This is safe practice in patients with lymphoma who are undergoing chemotherapy, and in children who are in the induction phase for treatment of acute leukaemia.

TABLE 3.3 Common infecting organisms

Bacteria, Gram positive	Staphylococcus aureus
	Streptococcus
	Listeria
	Nocardia asteroides
	Mycobacterium tuberculosis
Bacteria, Gram negative	Enterobacteriaceae
	Pseudomonas aeruginosa
	Legionella
	Bacteroides
Fungi	Candida
	Aspergillus
	Cryptococcus
	Pneumocystis carinii
	Histoplasma capsulatum
Parasites	Toxoplasma gondii
	Strongyloides stercoralis
Viruses	Herpes—h. simplex. h. zoster, CMV, EBV
	Hepatitis B and C
	HIV (from blood, very rarely)

PAIN MANAGEMENT

In a patient's mind, pain is almost always associated with the diagnosis of cancer and it is often feared more than death itself. Over 70% of patients with cancer have moderate to severe pain, but over 85% can obtain excellent control with conventional analgesia. Pain may be acute, chronic or incidental and may be differentiated into somatic, neuropathic or visceral types. When the aetiology of the pain has been established, it may be treated pharmacologically, with radiotherapy, chemotherapy, palliative surgery, nerve blocks or by TENS.

Prior to prescribing analgesia, the following points should be addressed.

History Pain site, quality, exacerbating/relieving factors, temporal pattern, duration, associated symptoms, trend (deteriorating with time?), effect on daily life and psychology, response to previous analgesic efforts.

Examination Search for possible mass effects, swelling, inflammation/infection, ulceration, muscle wasting, dermatome distribution, reflex abnormalities, sensory loss and, where appropriate, gait and fundoscopy.

Investigations Renal and liver function tests • Plain X-rays • Bone scan • ultrasound/Doppler scan • CT scan • MR scan • Nerve conduction tests • Occasionally endoscopy.

The choice of treatment modality depends on the conclusion reached using the above procedures.

Analgesics

Non-opiate analgesics
- Simple analgesics (e.g. paracetamol) taken regularly: effective against milder pain.
- NSAIDs (e.g. diclofenac): effective for bone or liver capsule pain. **NB**: will require H_2 antagonist if thrombocytopenic tendency.
- Steroids: helpful in liver capsular pain (e.g. prednisolone 30 mg daily); reduce headache from raised ICP (e.g. dexamethasone 16 mg daily).
- Intermediate analgesics (e.g. co-proxamol, codeine phosphate): often effective when paracetamol alone fails.
- Others (e.g. carbamazepine, dothiepin, flecainide, amitriptyline): helpful in postherpetic neuralgia and other neuropathic pain.

Opiates
Reassure patient that in correct dosage these are not associated with 'becoming a zombie', addiction or imminent death. Most opiate-related side-effects (e.g. nausea, constipation) can be prevented or relieved. Laxatives should always be prescribed with opiates.

- Codeine phosphate—normally considered with the 'intermediate' group of analgesics; metabolized to morphine.
- Sevredol/morphine elixir—tablet/liquid preparation for regular use in moderate to severe pain.
- MST—sustained release morphine for twice daily oral administration.
- Pethidine—usually less effective than above options; rapid but short-lived effect.
- Methadone—occasionally useful alternative to morphine; beware accumulation.
- Fentanyl—100 times stronger than morphine; transdermal patches are convenient, effective and cause less constipation.

Continuous analgesic delivery
Continuous administration of analgesics through slow-release oral, transdermal or subcutaneous delivery to prevent pain breakthrough is more effective than intermittent dosing according to immediate need.

Allow slow low-dose delivery of diamorphine by subcutaneous needle attached to a syringe pump (e.g. 10 mg over 12 h) to achieve good pain control and a low incidence of side-effects.

Chemotherapy
- Bone pain secondary to leukaemia—responds well.
- Tumours where response is associated with reduction in pressure from growth.
- Even where there is no objective evidence of tumour response (e.g. non-small cell lung cancer).

Radiotherapy
- Single-fraction radiotherapy to site of bone pain—effective in > 70% of cases.
- Shrinkage of a tumour mass (e.g. malignant nodes) to relieve pain.
- Back or leg pain secondary to spinal cord compression—responds to fractionated radiotherapy.
- Lowering of ICP from irradiation of cerebral metastases to improve headache.

Surgery
- Skin and soft tissue—painful masses or nodes can be treated by surgery or by radiotherapy (see above).
- Bone—stabilization of collapsed vertebrae to alleviate back pain.
- Nerve—decompression of a spinal cord compression to alleviate nerve root irritation.

Nerve block
In severe, intractable nerve pain, may be effective when performed by an experienced anaesthetist.

TENS

Small-voltage electrical nerve stimulation to relieve neuralgic pain.
Physiotherapists are experienced in the use of TENS, as are anaesthetists
who specialize in pain control.

PLEURAL EFFUSION

In cancer medicine, a pleural effusion is usually caused by pleural involvement
by tumour, e.g. breast cancer. Other causes include transdiaphragmatic spread
of ascites, hypoalbuminaemia and pulmonary embolism. Depending on the
amount of fluid, its rate of accumulation and the presence of underlying lung
disease, the patient may be relatively asymptomatic or bedbound.

Treatment of the effusion relates entirely to symptoms and should not be
initiated unless necessary. Note that pleural fluid may contain malignant cells
and can aid in both diagnosis and staging of a neoplasm.

Making the diagnosis
- CXR.
- Thoracic ultrasound—will inform whether or not the fluid is loculated.
- Cytology.
- Protein content (exudate—contains > 40 g/L protein).

Treatment
1. Insert percutaneous tube under local anaesthetic (narrow-gauge catheters
   are usually as effective and are less traumatic than wider-gauge cannulae).
2. Drain slowly (500 ml/30 min).
3. When drained to dryness, clamp tube and perform pleurodesis with
   bleomycin 60 mg injected through the drain.
4. Encourage the patient to roll into different positions to ensure adequate
   pleural spread of the sclerosing agent.
5. Unclamp tube after a minimum of 6 h and remove chest drain. The patient
   is very likely to spike a high pyrexia in the 12 h following bleomycin
   pleurodesis.

Tetracycline pleurodesis is an alternative, but is often very painful.
Lignocaine 20 ml should be added to the injection.

Problems
- Loculated effusion—drainage of pockets under ultrasound control may be
  possible; pleurodesis will not be effective.
- Pneumothorax—drain if > 30%; if smaller, aspirate if possible.
- Lung does not drain to dryness—attach Roberts' pump and apply suction
  overnight or longer; repeat CXR daily.

- Pain at site of cannula insertion—if simple / intermediate analgesics or local anaesthetic cream / infiltration is not helpful, the drain may have to be removed.
- Recurrent, symptomatic effusion—refer to cardiothoracic surgeon for possible surgical pleurodesis or insertion of pleuroperitoneal shunt.

RADIATION ENTERITIS

Radiation-induced inflammation of the bowel occurs as a function of the volume of bowel irradiated and the radiation dose. Prior abdominal surgery increases the likelihood of radiation enteritis. It is unusual for acute radiation enteritis to become severe enough to require interruption of radiotherapy.

Cancers where the radiation field encompasses bowel include: • uterine cervix • uterine body • bladder • abdominal lymphoma • ovary • kidney • testicular tumours • stomach • pancreas • prostate.

ACUTE RADIATION ENTERITIS

This occurs during therapy and over the subsequent few weeks. It manifests as ileitis, colitis or proctitis, with abdominal pain, diarrhoea and tenesmus with occasional mucus or blood.

Management
- Relieve abdominal discomfort with agents which give form to a fluid stool (e.g. isogel granules).
- In more severe cases give medication to reduce bowel motility.
- In rare cases where peritonism or signs of intestinal perforation develop, radiotherapy is stopped and surgical management proceeds as for perforated abdominal viscus (see p. 35).

LATE RADIATION ENTERITIS

Onset is 6–24 months post radiotherapy.

Symptoms
- Colicky abdominal pain.
- Intermittent diarrhoea, occasionally with blood and mucus.
- May cause strictures giving rise to intestinal obstruction.
- Fistula formation is very unusual in the absence of advanced malignant disease.

Management

Many cases settle with conservative management and appropriate dietary precautions. A small proportion require resection of the involved bowel segment.

SECOND MALIGNANCY

The risk of patients developing a second primary tumour years later is due to the irreversible genetic damage caused by some chemotherapies. It is not possible to predict which patients are at highest risk, but several drugs are implicated (Tables 3.4 & 3.5).

TABLE 3.4 Second primary tumour: risk factors

Malignancy	Hodgkin's disease
	testicular teratoma
	ovarian carcinoma
	breast cancer
	childhood malignancies
Non-malignant conditions	prolonged immunosuppression with cytotoxics in e.g. organ/tissue transplant, rheumatoid arthritis

TABLE 3.5 Drugs associated with carcinogenicity

Definite	Possible (in vitro studies)	No evidence of carcinogenicity
Chlorambucil	Actinomycin-D	Cytosine arabinoside
Cyclophosphamide	Bleomycin	5-fluorouracil
Etoposide	Cisplatin	Methotrexate
Melphalan	Doxorubicin	
Nitrogen mustard	Vinca alkaloids	
Nitrosourea		
Procarbazine		
Thiotepa		

Time-lapse post treatment • Leukaemias — 6–10 years • Lymphomas — ≥ 15 years • Solid tumours — > 15 years, with no apparent time limit on duration of risk.

Features of treatment associated with high risk • High doses • Low doses chronically delivered • Combination chemotherapy – irradiation • Combination of several 'high-risk' drugs.

Mechanisms

1. Drugs which interact with cellular DNA may not kill the cell but may induce sublethal changes which can be passed on to progeny and can be associated with later changes to the malignant phenotypes. Hence DNA-intercalating agents are 'high risk' while antimetabolites, e.g. 5-FU, are considered to be non-carcinogenic.
2. Chronic immunosuppression prevents the body's immune system from monitoring the production of abnormal cells during cell division. This leads to a failure to identify or attack the small cancers which may frequently develop in the normal person.

Implications

Solid tumours are treated with the drugs which best induce a remission, since the immediate problem of the cancer is paramount. Higher-risk agents, e.g. alkylating agents, should be used with caution in the adjuvant setting or in neoadjuvant treatment of potentially curable tumours.

Suspected carcinogenicity cannot be proven until the drug has been used in thousands of patients over a period of at least 20 years. Regular analysis of cytogenetics in samples from previously treated patients may identify early high-risk changes which can be reversed. However, this possibility has not yet been explored.

SYNDROME OF INAPPROPRIATE ADH

In cancer patients, the syndrome of inappropriate ADH (SIADH) may be caused by:

- increased secretion of ADH from a peptide-secreting tumour (e.g. SCLC, carcinoid, pancreatic adenocarcinoma, lymphoma, leukaemia)
- drugs (e.g. high-dose cyclophosphamide, ifosfamide, vincristine)
- associated factors (e.g. pneumonia, intracranial lesions).

Making the diagnosis
Effects of low serum sodium • Headache • Weakness • Confusion • Drowsiness • Seizure.

Investigations • U+Es • $Na^+ < 130$ mmol/L and K^+ normal • Osmolalities with urine > plasma • Continued excretion of urinary Na^+.

Management
- Restrict fluid intake to < 1 litre daily (watch U+Es).
- Demeclocycline 0.6–1.2 g daily.
- Treat underlying cause where appropriate.

Infusion of hypertonic saline is only rarely necessary, and the consequent rapid sudden electrolyte shifts over less than 48 h may initially increase the patient's confusion and irritability.

STOMA MANAGEMENT

A carelessly constructed stoma can cause life-long misery. The keys to success are:

- careful preoperative planning and counselling
- involvement of a specialist stoma care nurse
- familiarity with the range of modern appliances and stoma care products. If the hospital does not have a specialist nurse, stoma product manufacturers employ nurse advisors to help with practical problems.

Constructing a stoma
- Avoid paramedian incisions at laparotomy as they may compromise the siting of any stoma at the ideal position.
- The stoma incision should pass through the rectus sheath as this has a lower risk of paracolostomy hernia than a more laterally sited incision.
- The aperture must easily accommodate two fingers.
- The bowel must be of a comfortable length to avoid tension.
- The mesentery must not be twisted, stretched or compromised.
- The lateral space should either be
  — sutured closed (usually best for a colostomy) or
  — left wide open (usually best for an ileostomy).

Postoperative problems
Dusky colour in early postoperative period Discolouration is common in the first few days, but check for signs of full-thickness bowel infarction:

- circumferential blue/black colour
- no pink mucosa seen on digital or proctoscopic examination
- bowel retraction
- localised peritonitis.

Colostomy stenosis This late complication usually arises because of bowel ischaemia and retraction not severe enough to cause early peritonitis. Revisionary surgery requires re-laparotomy.

Colostomy prolapse This is particularly common with loop colostomies. Revisionary surgery may require re-laparotomy.

Paracolostomy hernia These may occasionally strangulate, but more often they cause symptoms through faecal distension which can be relieved by enemas.

Crevices or folds that cause appliances to fit badly.

THROMBOCYTOPENIA

Thrombocytopenia is mild when the platelet count is $< 150 \times 10^{12}/L$, moderate at $< 100 \times 10^{12}/L$ and severe at $< 50 \times 10^{12}/L$. Following standard or (especially) high-dose chemotherapy, platelet count may drop to $< 10 \times 10^{12}/L$. Patients with acute leukaemia or bone marrow infiltration with tumour are at risk of severe thrombocytopenia.

Patients should be warned to have FBC as soon as possible if they notice very easy bruising or red (petechial) haemorrhage around the ankles. Warfarin should be discontinued in patients who have been anticoagulated for a previous DVT.

Management
- Observation—for thrombocytopenia $< 20 \times 10^{12}/L$.
- Platelet transfusion recommended only for:
  — active bleeding (epistaxis, haemoptysis, haematemesis, haemorrhoids)
  — sepsis (in case of platelet consumption).
- Transfusion—usually recommended if the total platelet count is $< 10 \times 10^{12}/L$, or if $< 20 \times 10^{12}/L$ and packed cell transfusion is required.
- If a patient has a rigor during a platelet transfusion:
  — transfusion should be stopped
  — hydrocortisone 100 mg IV and chlorpheniramine 5 mg IV should be given
  — give next platelet transfusion through a filter to sift out white cell fragments.
- Occasionally, it may be necessary to tissue-type the patient to allow delivery of matched platelets and prevent further platelet reactions. Daily platelet counts are required to ensure that the increment post transfusion is maintained.
- Interleukin 3 (IL-3) is one of several growth factors currently under investigation for the ability to stimulate thrombocytes.

VENOUS ACCESS

Patients requiring chemotherapy, IV nutrition, bone marrow transplantation, repeated blood product administration, etc., may require prolonged venous access.

Peripheral venous access
The main principles of giving chemotherapy via peripheral veins are:

- Avoid side of disease in carcinoma of breast (risk of lymphoedema).
- Avoid antecubital fossa.
- Flush cannula through with saline, get good flash-back, give chemotherapy into running drip.
- If cytotoxic drug extravasates
  — stop chemotherapy infusion immediately
  — flush with normal saline
  — remove drip
  — apply ice
  — inform consultant.

Central venous access
Particularly useful for patients receiving:

- cytotoxic drugs associated with local tissue necrosis in the event of extravascular extravasation, e.g. adriamycin
- intermittent courses of chemotherapy over a prolonged period of time.

Tunnelled central line
A central venous catheter may be inserted:

- by percutaneous puncture (e.g. Seldinger technique).
- operatively into the subclavian vein or an internal jugular vein.

The catheter is tunnelled percutaneously for several cm so that the point of skin entry is at a distance from the point of central vein entry, to minimize the risk of catheter sepsis.

Central venous catheter with subcutaneous port
As an alternative to a tunnelled central line, a subcutaneous port may be attached to a central venous catheter entering the subclavian, internal jugular or even the femoral vein. Instead of an external catheter, it has a plastic dome that allows multiple percutaneous needle insertions.

MANAGING SPECIFIC TUMOURS

GASTROINTESTINAL TUMOURS

CARCINOMA OF THE OESOPHAGUS

Carcinomas of the upper and middle thirds of the oesophagus are usually SCCs, but in the lower third, over half are adenocarcinomas invading upwards from the cardia of the stomach or perhaps arising in 'ectopic' or dysplastic gastric mucosa (Barrett's oesophagus). There is a huge geographical variation in incidence. It is the leading cause of cancer death in China, but accounts for only 1–2% in the West.

Risk factors
These include: • alcohol • tobacco • opium tar • nutritional deficiencies—vitamin A, vitamin C, riboflavin • associated with chronic iron and vitamin deficiency in the Plummer–Vinson (Patterson–Kelly) syndrome (rare and decreasing) • tylosis (autosomal dominant condition of palmar and plantar hyperkeratosis)—45% lifetime risk of oesophageal cancer.

Making the diagnosis
Signs and symptoms • Dysphagia ± weight loss • Recurrent chest infections due to repeated aspiration of oesophageal contents.

Investigations
• Endoscopy—allows biopsy.
• Barium swallow—enables estimation of tumour length.

Either procedure may be performed for diagnosis, but both investigations should be performed as they give complementary information.

• CT scan—to look for spread into lymph nodes, mediastinum, lungs or liver. CT may give important information about resectability, but does not always accurately correlate with resectability.
• Mediastinoscopy—generally considered to be too invasive for this tumour type.
• Laparoscopy—useful to exclude peritoneal disease not visualized by CT scan.
• Surgical exploration—may be justified in younger patients with mediastinal lymphadenopathy (they may be reactive nodes).
• Endoscopic ultrasound—increasingly used to assess degree of local and nodal involvement.

Treatment

The first decision to be made is whether to treat the patient with curative or palliative intent. Factors to be considered include:

- presence of unequivocal metastatic disease on imaging or at laparoscopy
- patient age and performance status.

Curative intent

Surgery Resection is probably still the best approach for younger patients without evidence of distant spread. Methods of oesophagectomy include:

1. McKeown's operation—involves laparotomy, thoracotomy and cervical incision and an anastomosis of stomach to cervical oesophagus in the neck.
2. Ivor Lewis operation—involves laparotomy and thoracotomy and an anastomosis of stomach to upper oesophagus in the chest.
3. Thoraco-abdominal approach—involves single incision through left upper abdomen, diaphragm and chest and an anastomosis of stomach to upper oesophagus in the chest.
4. Transhiatal—involves laparotomy and cervical incision with blunt dissection of the thoracic oesophagus, lifting a gastric pedicle into the neck for a cervical anastomosis.
5. Laparoscopic-assisted—similar to the transhiatal operation, but using laparoscopic instruments for the thoracic mobilisation.

Radiotherapy Probably the treatment of choice for most SCCs of the upper and middle oesophagus, since this avoids the operative mortality of surgery and gives similar survival. No consensus exists as to the value of combining surgery with adjuvant radiotherapy. Preoperative radiotherapy has been assessed by randomized trial and does not appear to improve resection rates or survival. Several groups use postoperative radiotherapy to reduce local recurrence (a major cause of death) but the relative benefit of this approach compared to surgery alone is unknown.

Chemotherapy Can be effective in both SCC and adenocarcinoma, e.g. ECF (see Carcinoma of the stomach, pp. 70–72), and is being evaluated by several centres, particularly within the neoadjuvant setting. For SCC the chemotherapy – radiation combination has proven benefit over either modality alone.

Palliative intent

Treatment needs to be tailored to the individual patient according to the predominant symptoms and the local availability of the options.

1. Radiotherapy by external beam or intracavitary technique—a good option for squamous cell and some adenocarcinomas.

2. Intubation, e.g. using an endoscopically placed stent—particularly useful for the treatment of tracheo-oesophageal fistula.
3. Laser therapy—allows excellent palliation of dysphagia caused by exophytic tumours.

There is rarely any place for oesophageal resection as a palliative procedure.

Prognosis
Overall 4% 5-year survival

Patients who survive oesophageal resection Approximately 20% 5-year survival. Postoperative mortality of oesophagectomy should be < 10% but is often higher, especially for tumours of the upper and middle thirds.

CARCINOMA OF THE STOMACH

Gastric cancer is the second most frequently occurring tumour type worldwide. It is the leading cause of cancer death in Japan and the fourth most common tumour in Europe. Although the incidence is decreasing overall, there is an increase in tumours of the proximal stomach and oesophagogastric junction.

Risk factors
- Age—commoner in older people.
- Diet and nutrition
  - associated with high intake of nitrates, salt and complex carbohydrates
  - linked with low intake of fresh fruits and greens.
- Associated with multifocal chronic gastritis and (rarely) autoimmune gastritis.
- Linked to gastric infection with *H. pylori.*
- More common in people of Blood Group A.

Staging (→ Table 4.1)

TABLE 4.1 Staging carcinoma of the stomach	
Laparotomy	The 'gold standard' for assessing degree of local and distant invasion
Endoscopic ultrasonography	Enables tumour depth to be measured
CT scanning	Enables involvement of both adjacent structures and metastases to be assessed

Preoperative staging by CT scan and laparoscopy are increasing in relevance as alternative treatment modalities are investigated. (Historically, intensive preoperative staging has been considered inappropriate since the majority underwent surgical staging at laparotomy.)

Making the diagnosis

Signs and symptoms • Dysphagia • Dyspepsia • Anorexia, weight loss • Epigastric 'fullness' • Iron-deficiency anaemia.

Investigations • Endoscopy and biopsy or brushings to investigate dyspepsia — successful in 95% of cases • Barium meal • Endoscopic screening to diagnose tumours at an early stage (30% as a result of screening programme in Japan compared with 1% in Britain).

Histology

The tumours are almost invariably adenocarcinoma:

- intestinal (results in polypoidal tumours)
- diffuse (results in linitis plastica).

There is poor correlation between histological grade and prognosis. The best prognosis is seen with 'early gastric cancer' in which the carcinoma is confined to the mucosa and submucosa — a lesion more commonly found in Japan as a result of population screening.

Treatment

Surgery The mainstay of gastric cancer treatment (approximately 80% of patients in UK). • Radical distal (partial) gastrectomy for distal tumours • Total gastrectomy with or without oesophagectomy for mid- and proximal cancers • The role of extended lymph node dissection is currently being investigated in a randomized UK trial • Palliative resection or bypass may be useful in cases where radical surgery is impossible.

Chemotherapy Of no proven benefit in the adjuvant setting, although there is an indication that mitomycin-C may improve survival. Neoadjuvant chemotherapy is now a feasible option: responses of up to 80% are reported with combination treatment, e.g. epirubicin, cisplatin and continuous infusion 5-FU (ECF). All patients treated with neoadjuvant chemotherapy should be included in a formal trial until conclusive results are obtained. In advanced disease, the standard FAMTX regimen (5-FU, adriamycin and methotrexate) is effective in 40% of patients and can improve median survival by 9 months when compared with best supportive care.

Radiotherapy There is no good evidence to suggest that radiotherapy is of significant benefit as an adjunct to surgery. The role of radiotherapy in palliation of unresectable tumours is restricted by its associated significant toxicity. Studies are under way to assess the efficacy of intraoperative radiotherapy to the gastric bed. In addition, there is evidence to suggest that irradiation may be more effective if delivered with radiosensitizing chemotherapy, e.g. 5-FU.

Prognosis

Early diagnosis and surgery 95% 5-year survival (Japan)

Patients who undergo surgery 55% 5-year survival with improved selection and operating techniques

Locally advanced disease (involving regional nodes) • Median survival 5 months postoperatively • No survivors at 2 years

Diffuse tumours These have a worse prognosis than tumours of intestinal histology

CARCINOMA OF THE PANCREAS

Pancreatic carcinoma accounts for approximately 20% of deaths from gastrointestinal cancer, and is increasing in incidence. This tumour type is associated with smoking. 66% of tumours occur in the anatomical head. Approximately 85% are advanced locally at the time of diagnosis, with metastatic disease present in 50% of cases.

Staging

In patients of good performance status with no radiological or clinical evidence of metastatic disease or portal vein involvement, radical resection may be considered. Cure is only possible in these circumstances.

Making the diagnosis

Signs and symptoms Tumours often present late. Symptoms, which are often non-specific, include: • back pain • abdominal pain • anorexia • weight loss • fever • jaundice (often indicative of advanced disease).

Investigations • Ultrasound • CT scanning • ERCP • Tumour marker CA19.9 > 2000 is suggestive of pancreatic primary.

Histology

The histological types are: • ductal adenocarcinoma (80%)
• cystadenocarcinomas • lymphoma • neuroendocrine • small cell
• undifferentiated.

Treatment

Surgery
• Radical resection (Whipple's procedure, pancreaticoduodenectomy), with or without pyloric preservation and lymph node dissection, carries high operative morbidity and mortality of about 10%, but offers the only real prospect for cure. There is no evident benefit of performing extended lymphadenectomy.

- Surgical biliary bypass (choledochojejunostomy, cholecystojejunostomy), prophylactic gastroenterostomy or endoscopic / percutaneous biliary decompression may be performed if definitive surgery is precluded by the extent of the tumour.

Chemotherapy There is no proven benefit of adjuvant chemotherapy in this disease. In advanced disease, two studies have demonstrated improved survival for patients treated with combination therapy using 5-FU, adriamycin and mitomycin-C (FAM) when compared with best supportive care — median survival 8 vs 3.5 months.

Radiotherapy There is evidence of improved results if chemotherapy is combined with radiotherapy in pancreatic cancer, but trials to confirm earlier results are still ongoing. Adjuvant external beam radiotherapy remains unproven. Some centres are evaluating intraoperative radiotherapy in this setting. In advanced disease radiotherapy is associated with significant gastrointestinal upset and this limits its role in palliation.

Prognosis
Resectable 5–10% 5-year survival postoperatively; 25% 5-year survival with improved selection and operating techniques

Overall 3–5% 5-year survival after diagnosis

CARCINOMA OF THE COLON AND RECTUM

Carcinoma of the colon and rectum is the third most common cause of cancer death in the UK. The incidence is increased in genetic syndromes, e.g. familial adenomatous polyposis, and in people with inflammatory bowel disease. These tumours are associated with high-fat, low-fibre diets. Low doses of aspirin may have a protective action.

The rate of relapse is 30%, with a mortality rate of > 50% by 5 years. Early diagnosis by 3–5-yearly screening by flexible sigmoidoscopy may be effective in people > 50 years of age.

Staging (→ Table 4.2)

TABLE 4.2 Staging carcinoma of colon/rectum: modified Duke's criteria	
A	Tumour limited to mucosa and submucosa
B1	Tumour reaching but not penetrating serosa
B2	Tumour through serosa to peritoneal cavity/contiguous organ
C	Spread to local lymph nodes
D	Metastases present

Making the diagnosis

Colorectal cancer is localized at diagnosis in 70% of cases.

Signs and symptoms: colon • Alteration in bowel habit • Rectal bleeding • Iron-deficiency anaemia • Abdominal discomfort • Intestinal obstruction or perforation (advanced disease).

Signs and symptoms: rectum • Rectal bleeding • Tenesmus • Feeling of incomplete bowel emptying.

Investigations • Perform digital rectal examination • Faecal occult blood test • Sigmoidoscopy ± colonoscopy ± barium enema. *If tumour is confirmed*: • CXR and abdominal CT scan or liver ultrasound • FBC • Chemistry (liver function tests) and carcinoembryonic antigen (CEA) should be checked.

Treatment

Radical surgical excision • Abdominoperineal resection for low rectal carcinoma • Resection with end-to-end anastomosis in upper rectal or colon cancer, with confirmation of clearance of all tumour by histologically clear resection margins recommended.

Adjuvant chemotherapy and radiotherapy 5-FU and levamisole given for 1 year reduce both relapse rate (by 41%) and death rate (by 33%) from Duke's C colon carcinoma. Alternative modulation of 5-FU with levamisole and continuous infusion 5-FU are being evaluated in the adjuvant setting.

Radiotherapy may be administered pre- or postoperatively to reduce local relapse in cancer of the rectum, but no improvement in survival has been seen so far. Combination of 5-FU and radiotherapy in high-risk rectal tumour (Duke's B2, B3, C) is synergistic, in terms of preventing local relapse with associated reduction in systemic relapse and improvement in overall survival.

Local recurrence

This is a common problem with cancer of the rectum, involving pelvic sidewall, sacrum and adjacent bowel. True 'anastomotic' recurrence is rare. Treatment can be difficult.

Surgical clearance Should be attempted, particularly if obstructive symptoms are present.

Pelvic irradiation Should be considered particularly for control of pain.

Chemotherapy Achieves useful palliation in patients with unresectable, symptomatic local recurrence, who have already received full-dose radiotherapy.

Metastatic disease

The median survival after diagnosis of metastatic colorectal cancer is 6–8 months.

Surgery Hepatic resection may be feasible where there is a solitary or few peripherally situated hepatic metastases. 5-year survival ≤ 25%.

Chemotherapy The most effective single agent is 5-FU, which achieves a response rate of around 20%. Scheduling of 5-FU refers to the optimum mode of delivery of the drug. Because of the mode of action as an S-phase specific drug with a short half-life, infusional treatment was investigated and found to increase the response rate to 35%. Side-effects—myelosuppression and mucositis—are less common with infusional 5-FU although plantar-palmar erythema can develop and may cause skin peeling and ulceration, unless administration is interrupted.

Regional chemotherapy The delivery of intrahepatic chemotherapy, usually with 5-FU given via the hepatic artery, appears to give an improvement in response rates, but there is a risk of hepatitis from the chemotherapy in addition to the risk of complications from the indwelling catheter.

CARCINOMA OF THE ANUS

Anal cancer is a relatively rare disease, but it can affect young adults.

Risk factors
- Strong epidemiological link with receptive anal intercourse in homosexual males.
- Linked with the human papilloma virus (HPV).
- Progression of genital warts (condylomata accuminata) to invasive carcinoma is well recognized.

Staging (→ Table 4.3)

TABLE 4.3 Staging in anal carcinoma	
T1	< 2 cm
T2	> 2–5 cm
T3	> 5 cm
T4	Adjacent organ(s)
N1	Perirectal
N2	Unilateral internal iliac/inguinal
N3	Perirectal and inguinal, bilateral internal iliac/inguinal

Making the diagnosis
Signs and symptoms • Typically presents with anal discomfort or bleeding
• Rectal examination reveals an ulcer with induration of the surrounding
tissues • Inguinal node involvement may be present.

 An important feature of anal cancer that differentiates it from
carcinoma of the lower rectum is its ability to spread to the inguinal
lymph nodes in addition to perirectal and iliac lymph nodes.

Differential diagnosis • Bleeding, pain: 'piles' • Anal ulceration:
fissure-in-ano, primary syphilis, Crohn's disease • Perirectal and iliac
lymph node involvement: carcinoma of the lower rectum.

Investigations • Rectal examination • Biopsy under GA — gives important
information about the degree of local and nodal spread and distinguishes
carcinoma of the anal canal from adenocarcinoma of the lower rectum
invading downwards • Careful examination of the inguinal nodes
• FNAC of enlarged nodes.

Histology
- Anal marginal tumours—arise from the squamous epithelium of the
  anal margin below the anal valves.
- Cloacogenic (or basaloid) carcinoma—histological variant of anal
  margin tumour.
- Anal canal tumours—arise from the transitional zone of mixed epithelial
  types above the dentate line.

Treatment
Radiotherapy Radical radiotherapy, with or without chemotherapy, is now
the primary treatment of choice, and the majority of patients achieve a good
response.

- Anal canal preserved in the majority of cases.
- Typically both primary tumour and inguinal nodes encompassed by the
  radiotherapy field, often with a boost to the anal canal.

Chemotherapy Whether or not chemotherapy provides significant additional
benefit is still uncertain. Synchronous 5-FU and mitomycin C chemotherapy
is under evaluation.

Surgery Abdominoperineal resection (APR) with permanent colostomy is
reserved for patients who relapse after radiotherapy (< 10% of patients
treated). If < 50% reduction in tumour volume is achieved 6 weeks after
completion of treatment, consideration should be given to salvage surgery.
Wound healing is difficult following radiotherapy to the perianal tissues. It is

wise to bring a rectus abdominis myocutaneous flap down into the pelvic floor and perineum at the time of salvage APR.

Prognosis
With radiotherapy: 60% 5-year survival reported. Anal margin tumours tend to have a better prognosis.

CARCINOMA OF THE GALL BLADDER AND BILIARY TREE

Cholangiocarcinoma may affect any part of the biliary tree from the lower end of the common bile duct to the intrahepatic biliary radicles. It accounts for 0.8% of all malignant tumours and is less common than hepatocellular carcinoma. The commonest sites are (a) the gall bladder and (b) the confluence of the right and left hepatic ducts.

Making the diagnosis
- Obstructive jaundice is the commonest presenting symptom.
- Carcinoma of the gall bladder may be found incidentally at cholecystectomy for gall stones.

Treatment
Surgery The 30-day mortality rate for all surgical procedures is around 20–30%.

- Resection of intrahepatic or hilar lesion is rarely feasible.
- Biliary drainage is the priority of treatment, preferably by placing a stent across the tumour at ERCP or following PTC.
- Formal laparotomy should be performed to achieve wide excision of adjacent tissues for carcinoma found at laparoscopic cholecystectomy.
- Several operative techniques of biliary – enteric bypass have been described for unresectable cholangiocarcinoma and may occasionally be indicated if attempts at internal stenting are unsuccessful.

Radiotherapy Good additional palliation may be achieved by local radiotherapy, e.g. by using an intracavitary technique utilizing external stents.

Chemotherapy Recent combination chemotherapy, e.g. ECF, suggests that this tumour may also be chemosensitive.

Prognosis
- Median survival from diagnosis < 6 months.
- Survival may be prolonged with slow-growing hilar tumours if biliary drainage can be achieved.
- Wide surgical resection of carcinoma of the gall bladder diagnosed incidentally at the time of cholecystectomy for stones can result in a curative outcome.

HEPATOCELLULAR CARCINOMA

Primary hepatocellular carcinoma (HCC) is rare in Western countries, but in many parts of Africa and Asia it is the most common cancer. The tumour may arise as a solitary mass, but more commonly there are multiple scattered tumour nodules.

Risk factors

Linked to hepatitis B virus—carriers have up to 100-fold increased relative risk. Diet—aflatoxin from mouldy food may be contributory factor in Africa and Asia. Associated with alcoholic cirrhosis in the West.

Making the diagnosis

Signs and symptoms
- In low-incidence areas, symptoms are often insidious:
  — general deterioration in the health of a known cirrhotic.
- In high-incidence areas:
  — right upper quadrant pain
  — abdominal distension due to hepatomegaly
  — ascites.
- Occasionally, HCC presents with:
  — major intraperitoneal haemorrhage
  — systemic manifestations, e.g. hypoglycaemia or hypercalcaemia.
- Raised serum alpha-fetoprotein (about 80%):
  — marginally raised values seen in viral hepatitis and in active cirrhosis
  — other causes of false positives: testicular and ovarian germ cell tumours, liver metastases from carcinoma of the stomach or pancreas.

Investigations • Liver ultrasound—detects majority of HCC • Hepatic arteriography for a solitary lesion—to confirm presence of tumour circulation and to assess arterial anatomy • Preliminary liver biopsy or cytology (if prothrombin time allows) under ultrasound, CT or laparoscopic control before resection • CT of the lungs before resection is contemplated. CT of the liver is unlikely to yield much extra information.

Treatment

Surgery Complete surgical excision is the only hope of cure, but resection is possible in < 10% of cases.

- Resection—feasible if lesion is confined to 1 segment or lobe, and remaining liver is not too cirrhotic.
- Resection of solitary lesions, with favourable arterial anatomy on arteriography—can prolong survival.

- Resection and liver transplantation—occasional long-term survivors have been reported.
- Selective hepatic artery embolisation—may be considered for symptomatic tumours as a means of producing temporary tumour necrosis.

Radiotherapy Has little to offer, even in palliation.

Chemotherapy Adriamycin, given IV or intra-arterially, may achieve worthwhile responses in alpha-fetoprotein levels or tumour volume. There is little point in persisting beyond 2 courses if no response is seen.

Prognosis
Overall 4% 5-year survival

Patients undergoing resection 15% 5-year survival. The best results are seen in resected cases who do not have cirrhosis, and patients with histological subtype—fibrolamellar variant.

CARCINOMA OF THE AMPULLA

Carcinoma of the ampulla of Vater is defined as a carcinoma arising within the distal common bile duct, distal pancreatic duct, ampulla or adjacent duodenal mucosa. It tends to have a better prognosis than carcinoma of the pancreas largely because it presents early with obstructive jaundice, while still only a few millimetres in diameter. The ratio of pancreatic to ampullary carcinoma is 10:1.

Making the diagnosis
Signs and symptoms > 10% of cases have undergone elective gall bladder surgery within 4 years of the diagnosis, either because gall stones are aetiological in the development of this disease or because symptoms have been wrongly attributed to incidental gall stones.

Investigations • Typically, ultrasound simply shows dilated common bile duct • ERCP, the best means of diagnosis, should always be performed in cases of jaundice where ultrasound and CT scan have failed to demonstrate a pancreatic mass.

Treatment
Surgery The treatment options are similar to those discussed for carcinoma of the pancreas.

- Radical surgery—offers the only hope of cure, but has a high operative mortality of about 10%.

- Partial duodenopancreatectomy developed by Whipple is the classical treatment, taking margins of uninvolved pancreas and duodenum.
- Non-surgical palliative biliary bypass (e.g. endoscopic placement of stent) is often a better alternative but:
  — denies the patient the opportunity for cure
  — is associated with some morbidity and mortality.
- In the elderly, preferable options are
  — endoscopic sphincterotomy alone, or
  — endoscopic stent placement or
  — local excisional surgery.

Prognosis

Overall survival 3% at 5 years

Successful resection About 25% at 5 years.

BREAST CARCINOMA

The highest incidence of breast cancer is found in England and Wales, closely followed by the rest of the UK, the USA and affluent European countries. The incidence is rising at a rate of over 1% per annum, the current overall lifetime incidence being over 1 in 12 with 3.5% of all women dying of this disease.

Risk factors (→ Table 4.4)

TABLE 4.4 Risk factors for breast cancer in women

Risk factor	Compared with	Typical relative risk
1st-degree relative > 60 years	No 1st-degree relative affected	1.4
1st-degree relative < 60 years	No 1st-degree relative affected	2
2 1st-degree relatives	No 1st-degree relative affected	4
Age 11–13 at menarche	Aged 16 years at menarche	1.3
Nulliparous	1st child at < 20 years	1.9
1st child at > 30 years	1st child at < 20 years	1.9
Atypical hyperplasia	No previous breast biopsy	4
HRT (current use)	Never used	1.3

The risk for women with a family history of breast cancer rises even further if a 1st-degree relative has had bilateral breast cancer, or if the disease appeared before the age of 40 years.

HRT and breast cancer

- There is no current consensus
- There is some evidence to link HRT with an increased risk of developing breast cancer:
  — restricted to prolonged use > 8 years
  — seen mainly in women > 60 years
  — appears to be lost as soon as HRT is stopped.
- In counselling women about the risk of breast cancer, it is important to balance this against the reduced risks of dying of myocardial infarction or stroke
- For women with an established diagnosis of breast cancer, there is no good evidence to suggest that HRT is detrimental to subsequent prognosis

Screening
- \> 50 years of age:
  - — regular screening mammography reduces breast cancer mortality by up to 25% in a screened population assuming > 70% compliance
  - — in the UK, two-view screening mammography is offered to all women 50–64 years of age every 3 years.
- 40–50 years of age:
  - — screening mammography not yet convincingly demonstrated to improve survival.
- Screening of high-risk women should probably commence at 40 years of age.
- \< 40 years of age:
  - — avoid screening mammography
  - — use mammography for assessment of symptomatic lump.
- Regular breast self-examination:
  - — probably results in tumours being diagnosed at a size more easily treated with breast-conserving surgery
  - — may have some marginal influence on survival.

Making the diagnosis
Signs and symptoms • Breast lump • Breast pain • Nipple retraction • Nipple discharge • Axillary lump • Peau d'orange • Inflammation.

Investigations • FNAC • Ultrasound • Mammography • TruCut biopsy.

The key to diagnosis is 'triple assessment' involving:
- examination • breast imaging • cytology or needle biopsy.

Staging
The TNM system is described in Table 4.5. For practical purposes the single most important staging information is axillary lymph node status.

- 'Node-negative' (stage I) has a much better prognosis than 'node-positive' (stage II).
- The lowest-risk disease is node-negative with tumours < 1 cm in diameter or of low-grade special histological type.
- The highest-risk disease is node-positive with > 10 nodes involved and high-grade histology.

Carcinoma of breast: chemoprevention
An interesting finding from large multicentre trials of adjuvant tamoxifen has been the reduced risk of contralateral breast cancer in patients receiving this drug. This has led to the suggestion that tamoxifen may similarly prevent breast cancer developing in women at high risk of the disease, by virtue of some of the risk factors outlined above. This is currently being investigated by randomized double-blind trial in several centres.

TABLE 4.5 Summary of TNM system

Stage T1	≤ 2 cm		
A	≤ 0.5 cm		
B	> 0.5–1 cm		
C	> 1–2 cm		
Stage T2	**> 2–5 cm**		
Stage T3	**> 5 cm**		
Stage T4	**Involvement of chest wall or skin**		
A	Involvement of chest wall		
B	Skin oedema or ulceration or satellite skin nodules in same breast		
C	A+B		
D	Inflammatory carcinoma		
Stage N1	**Movable axillary node on same side**	Stage pN1	
		A	Micrometastasis, i.e. ≤ 0.2 cm
		B	Metastasis
			i 1–3 nodes > 0.2–< 2 cm
			ii ≥ 4 nodes > 0.2–< 2 cm
			iii Tumour extending through capsule, node < 2 cm
			iv Node ≥ 2 cm
Stage N2	**Fixed axillary node on same side**	Stage pN2	
Stage N3	**Internal mammary nodes on same side**	Stage pN3	

Histology

There are five major types of invasive breast carcinoma:

- Invasive ductal carcinoma (75%):
  — characteristically has the hard gritty consistency of an unripe pear when incised.
- Invasive lobular carcinoma (10%):
  — a more diffuse lesion but carries a similar risk of metastasis
  — more often multicentric and bilateral
  — more often metastasizes to meninges and serosal surfaces.
- Tubular, medullary and mucinous:
  — 'special types' which generally carry a better prognosis.

Ductal carcinoma in situ (DCIS)

- Pre-invasive type seen much more commonly since the introduction of routine screening mammography.
- Approximate 40% local recurrence rate following lumpectomy alone, half with invasive carcinoma.
- Mastectomy is associated with a 98% chance of cure, but many patients wish to have breast conservation.
- Complete local excision ± radiotherapy ± tamoxifen, with close surveillance of residual breast, is usual treatment.
- No consensus as to the best treatment.

Lobular carcinoma in situ (LCIS)

- Probably histological marker of increased risk rather than premalignant lesion.
- Carries 1% per annum risk of invasive breast cancer in either breast, usually invasive ductal rather than invasive lobular carcinoma.
- Observation as for women with other significant risk factors, e.g. strong family history.
- The role of radiotherapy or tamoxifen in LCIS is uncertain
  — women who are uncomfortable with their level of risk of developing invasive carcinoma may opt for bilateral prophylactic mastectomy.
- Women with LCIS are suitable for inclusion in a chemoprevention trial.

Treatment of invasive breast cancer

Early 'operable' breast cancer

Local Choice of treatment—survival rates equivalent—is usually based on technical factors such as multifocal involvement, involvement of the nipple or patient preference.

- Mastectomy (with or without reconstruction).
- Breast-conserving surgery combined with postoperative radiotherapy to the residual breast.

Axilla Axillary clearance or sampling are currently the preferred options because of the clinical importance of lymph node histology.

1. Radical axillary dissection ('clearance') for local control and staging information about node status. Radiotherapy to the axilla should not be given following clearance because of the high risk of lymphoedema.
2. Axillary node sampling (usually four lymph nodes) with selective axillary irradiation to node-positive women.
3. Axillary surgery can be avoided in patients with an in-situ or low-risk carcinoma (< 1 cm, well differentiated).

Systemic Adjuvant therapy is essential for the majority because of the risk of occult micrometastasis.

- Cytotoxic chemotherapy in premenopausal women and tamoxifen in postmenopausal women each reduces the relative risk of death by about 25% at 10 years.
- Combination cytotoxic chemotherapy and tamoxifen appears to give a marginal extra benefit in both premenopausal and postmenopausal women.
- Ovarian ablation is associated with a similar improvement in survival rates for premenopausal women and is used in some centres.

Locally advanced and inflammatory breast cancer
Systemic therapy is the priority. Surgery alone is unlikely to provide local control. There is also a high risk of metastatic disease. Initial treatment is chemotherapy/tamoxifen followed by radiotherapy and often mastectomy.

Local recurrence
In the residual breast Following breast-conserving treatments. Most require salvage mastectomy. Associated with impaired prognosis because it is an indication of biological aggressiveness, rather than because it leads to further opportunity for metastasis, i.e. it is a 'marker' rather than a 'determinant'.

Skin metastases Following mastectomy or breast-conserving surgery; can be treated by: • local excision • local radiation • hormone therapy • chemotherapy (particularly if associated with distant metastases).

Chest wall Optimum treatment usually depends on whether or not metastases can be identified at other sites. In the presence of metastatic disease—systemic therapy is the better option. In the absence of metastatic disease—consideration should be given to chest wall resection, which can be associated with prolonged survival.

Metastatic disease
Principles of management
- Intensive staging investigations during follow-up are inappropriate, since the early detection and treatment of asymptomatic distant metastases confer no survival benefit.
- The purpose of standard chemotherapy for metastatic disease is to palliate symptoms rather than to prolong survival.
- Patients with metastases in liver or lung should receive cytotoxic chemotherapy, e.g. CMF, MMM and adriamycin-based regimens.
- Bone metastases are more likely to respond to hormone manipulation using tamoxifen (if not previously exposed), LHRH-analogue (for premenopausal women) or a second-line hormonal agent such as megestrol or an aromatase inhibitor.

• Postmenopausal women may respond to hormone therapy for symptomatic metastases as the treatment of first choice. Visceral disease, e.g. liver, is normally an indication for chemotherapy.

Neoadjuvant therapy in primary breast cancer

Selection criteria
• Patients with large primary tumours (who would otherwise undoubtedly require mastectomy)
• Patients with high-risk disease, e.g. high-grade histology

Advantages of receiving cytotoxic chemotherapy 'up-front' before surgery or radiotherapy
• May allow preoperative shrinkage of the tumour, thus reducing the likelihood of mastectomy
• Enables assessment of chemo-responsiveness of the tumour to particular agents, thus theoretically allowing individualization of systemic therapy.

High dose chemotherapy
High dose chemotherapy involving a variety of drug combinations given at maximal dosage with subsequent peripheral blood stem cell infusion may be used for patients at very high risk, e.g. primary breast cancer with more than ten positive lymph nodes, or patients on first relapse with distant metastases. The drugs are usually given in sequential fashion to maximise response. Early results suggest that this approach gives better survival rates than conventional chemotherapy, but these regimens can be only be delivered in specialised centres able to cope with major pancytopenia-related complications. Some treatment-related deaths have occurred.

Endocrine therapy in breast cancer

Tamoxifen
• 60% response rates in metastatic or locally advanced disease.
• Well established in adjuvant setting for all postmenopausal women and for ER positive premenopausal women. Reduces relative risk of death by about 25%.
• Response may last many years.
• Occasional 'flare' of symptoms may occur during first month of treatment, e.g. pain from bone metastases, hypercalcaemia, spinal cord compression.
• Patients relapsing while on tamoxifen may occasionally show a tamoxifen withdrawal response.
• Patients relapsing after good initial response have a high chance of responding to second line endocrine therapy.

Gonadorelin analogues (e.g. zoladex)
- Cause reversible ovarian ablation.
- Under evaluation as adjuvant therapy in premenopausal women.
- Useful response rates in metastatic disease.

Aromatase inhibitors (e.g. lentaron, arimidex, aminoglutethimide)
- Postmenopausal women.
- Main role as second line endocrine therapy following relapse on tamoxifen.
- Newer agents have fewer side-effects than aminoglutethimide.
- Less weight gain than with progestogens.

Progestogens
Megestrol or Medroxyprogesterone acetate—alternative second line endocrine therapy. May cause weight gain through fluid retention or improvement in appetite.

UROLOGICAL TUMOURS

CARCINOMA OF THE KIDNEY

RENAL CELL CARCINOMA

Renal cell carcinoma (also known as 'Grawitz tumour') has a characteristic histological appearance of large clear cells. The tumour edge tends to be well demarcated and gives the false impression of being encapsulated, but the tumour frequently invades into perinephric fat and other tissues.

Making the diagnosis

Signs and symptoms • Classic triad: frank haematuria + loin pain + a loin mass • Occasionally: PUO, high-output cardiac failure (due to A–V shunts within tumour), hormonal effects, e.g. polycythaemia, hypercalcaemia or renin-mediated hypertension.

Investigations • IVU—usually makes diagnosis • Angiography and CT scan should also be performed to exclude a contralateral lesion and to look for evidence of renal vein involvement on the venous phase of angiography • Renal ultrasound.

Treatment

Primary tumour
Surgery
Radical nephrectomy Recommended for unilateral tumour, being prepared for resection of tumour extension along the renal vein into the inferior vena cava (IVC), together with a portion of IVC if necessary.

Partial nephrectomy If bilateral tumour or hypoplastic uninvolved kidney.

Some surgeons find that preoperative arterial embolization is useful in order to reduce vascularity, but this procedure causes considerable pain during the interval between embolisation and surgery.

Lung metastases
Spontaneous regression of a lung secondary following nephrectomy is a rare but well-documented phenomenon. Its incidence is less than the postoperative mortality rate associated with nephrectomy. Therefore, in the presence of metastases, nephrectomy should be restricted to those patients with local symptoms.

Systemic therapy The majority of patients with lung metastases have inoperable multiple deposits.

- Hormone therapy with Provera—widely used low-toxicity treatment, but response rates are low.
- Biological agents such as interferon or interleukin—can obtain better response rates but should be prescribed in the context of a clinical trial as the optimal regimen is as yet unknown. Better response rates are seen in patients with a prolonged disease-free interval.

Metastasectomy Surgical metastasectomy, perhaps even concurrently with nephrectomy, should be considered for patients with solitary lung metastasis, as prolonged survival is possible after such surgery. Best results are obtained for patients with 1–4 peripherally situated metastases who have a good performance status.

Prognosis
Following resection of primary tumour: 30–50% 5-year survival.

TRANSITIONAL CELL CARCINOMA (TCC) OF THE RENAL PELVIS AND URETER
The aetiology is similar to TCC of the bladder.

Making the diagnosis
Signs and symptoms • Typically presents with haematuria and ureteric colic • 50% per cent of cases are associated with TCC at other sites in the urothelium.

Investigations • IVU—often confirms diagnosis • Cystoscopy—to look at bladder mucosa and cannulate affected ureter • Cytology—specimens can be taken from affected ureter • Retrograde ureterography • Ureteroscopy.

Treatment
Surgery Radical nephroureterectomy is performed to remove the affected kidney together with the ureter and a cuff of bladder surrounding the ureteric orifice. This may involve 2 surgical incisions.

Radiotherapy Patients with positive resection margins may receive postoperative radiotherapy to the tumour bed.

Long-term follow-up
This involves check cystoscopy in a similar fashion to TCC of the bladder (see p. 91).

Prognosis
Overall 50% 5-year survival post radical nephroureterectomy.

CARCINOMA OF THE BLADDER

Bladder cancer accounts for over 5000 deaths each year in the UK. There is a male preponderance (3:1).

Carcinoma of bladder: natural history

- Non-invasive papillary tumours
  — 80% superficial non-invasive papillary tumours
  — may be single or multiple
  — 5–10% progress to invasive tumours
  — likelihood of progression increases as tumours become less differentiated (Grades II and III)

- Carcinoma in situ
  — can be multifocal
  — 30–50% progress to invasive disease
  — most recurrences within the first 2 years

- Invasive carcinoma
  — no previous history of superficial tumour in approximately 60% of patients
  — synchronous tumours may occur anywhere along the urothelial tract
  — lymphatic involvement
  — spread to perivesical, obturator, external, common iliac nodes
  — nodal disease in approximately 50% of patients with T3 tumours at the time of presentation

Risk factors

TCC Associated with tobacco smoking, exposure to aniline dyes (beta naphthylamine) and urinary stasis (7% occur in diverticula).

SCC Risk increased by *Schistosoma haematobium* infection.

Adenocarcinoma May appear in association with persistent urachal remnant.

Staging (→ Table 4.6)

TABLE 4.6 Carcinoma of bladder: staging	
Tis	Carcinoma in situ
Ta	Papillary non-invasive
T1	Invasion of lamina propria
T2	Superficial muscle invasion
T3a	Deep muscle invasion
T3b	Infiltrating perivesical fat
T4	Involvement of other organs, e.g. prostate, uterus, vagina
N1	Single lymph node < 2 cm
N2	Single or multiple < 5 cm
N3	> 5 cm

Making the diagnosis

Signs and symptoms Examination is frequently unremarkable.
- Common
  — painless haematuria.
- Less common
  — cystitis and urinary frequency
  — loin pain—may indicate an obstructed kidney
  — pelvic or low back pain—may herald pelvic organ infiltration or nodal disease.
- Advanced local or metastatic disease
  — general physical examination may reveal pallor from renal impairment or malignant cachexia
  — palpation of the abdomen may reveal a hydronephrotic kidney
  — rectal examination sometimes reveals a locally advanced tumour.

Investigations • FBC and biochemical profile • Urine cytology • IVU or abdominal ultrasound • Cystoscopy with EUA and biopsy • CT or MR scan.

Histology
- TCC: > 80%.
- SCC: 5%.
- Adenocarcinoma: 5%.
- Other cell types, including non-Hodgkin's lymphoma and soft tissue sarcomas: 5%.

Treatment

Superficial tumours
- Cystoscopic resection and regular cystoscopic follow-up.
- Intravesical chemotherapy (e.g. mitomycin) or BCG in cases of persistent multiple tumours.
- Cystectomy for carcinoma in situ, local recurrence.

Muscle-invasive carcinoma (T2/T3 – N0)
Treatment options:

- primary radiotherapy
- primary cystectomy
- partial cystectomy in selected cases.

Surgery Involves cystourethrectomy with either ileal urostomy or bladder reconstruction procedure.

Features favouring initial surgery • Carcinoma in situ • Carcinoma in a diverticulum • Reduced bladder capacity (< 200 ml) • Multiple tumours.

Radiotherapy Treatment planning is usually carried out using CT scan images of the pelvis. Treatment field may encompass the bladder alone or include the pelvic lymph nodes. Takes place over 3–6 weeks. Tumour dose 50–60 gray. Cystoscopic follow-up at 4–6-month intervals.

Chemotherapy The place of chemotherapy in the neoadjuvant setting is subject to ongoing clinical trials. A 30–40% response rate is seen in metastatic disease, most regimens including cisplatin or methotrexate.

Prognosis (→ Table 4.7)

TABLE 4.7 Carcinoma of the bladder: prognosis

Stage	5-year survival
T1	80%
T2	60%
T3	35%
T4	5%
	1-year survival
Nodal metastases	15%
Extranodal metastases	< 5%

Sequelae

Treatment-related Reduced bladder capacity following radiotherapy.

Disease-related Patients remain at risk of further tumours elsewhere in the urothelial tract. Close follow-up is essential.

PROSTATE CANCER

Prostate cancer is a disease of older men constituting the third most common male cancer in the UK, and the incidence is increasing. At presentation 20–30% are well-differentiated adenocarcinomas, 10% poorly differentiated and the remainder are moderately differentiated. Carcinomas arise in the peripheral zone of the prostate and tumours spread locally to involve the seminal vesicles. Bone metastases are common. Local progression, lymph node involvement and distant metastatic spread are associated with less well-differentiated tumours.

Risk factors
- Associated with circulating testosterone
  — not seen in castrated men
  — less frequent in liver cirrhotics.

- Reports of increased risk following vasectomy.
- Family history in a very small percentage of patients.

Staging (→ Table 4.8)

TABLE 4.8 Prostate cancer: staging	
T1	Incidental finding
a	< 3 microscopic foci
b	> 3 microscopic foci
T2	Presents clinically limited to the gland
a	< 1.5 cm with normal tissue on 3 sides
b	> 1.5 cm or involving more than 1 lobe
T3	Through capsule but not fixed
T4	Fixed or invades adjacent structures
N1	Single lymph node < 2 cm
N2	Single or multiple nodes < 5 cm
N3	> 5 cm

Making the diagnosis

Signs and symptoms
Asymptomatic disease:
- Post-mortem series have shown foci of well-differentiated prostate cancer in 30% of men over 75 years, indicating that prostatic cancer can run an indolent course.
- May present incidentally following TUR for BPH.
- Elevated serum prostatic specific antigen (PSA)—found on routine screening.

Symptomatic disease:
- Prostatic symptoms
  — reduced potency
  — urinary frequency + nocturia
  — poor stream
  — hesitancy
  — terminal dribbling.
- Perineal pain—indicates locally advanced disease.
- Pathological fracture or bone pain from metastatic disease—may be the first symptoms.
- Rarely, symptoms of nodal disease, e.g. unilateral or bilateral leg oedema.

Investigations • Physical examination—may be normal in early stage disease • Rectal examination typically reveals a hard irregular prostate; obliteration of the median sulcus with locally more advanced disease • FBC and biochemical profile • Serum PSA and acid phosphatase • IVU or abdominal ultrasound • Transrectal ultrasound • Cystourethroscopy with EUA and biopsy • Transrectal biopsy • Bone scan • CT or MR scan of abdomen and pelvis • Preoperative lymph node sampling (laparoscopic).

Treatment

Localized T1 well-differentiated carcinomas Non-intervention may be appropriate, particularly in an elderly man with a limited life expectancy.

Remaining localized tumours (T1 and T2) Can be treated with either radical prostatectomy or local radiotherapy. Radiotherapy is more commonly undertaken in the UK.

Surgery • TURP—relieves obstruction and provides histology • Radical prostatectomy including removal of the prostatic urethra, seminal vesicles, Denonvillier's fascia with lymph node dissection. Nerve-sparing procedures have greatly reduced the incidence of postoperative impotence.

Radiotherapy Usually external beam therapy using CT scan planning. Toxicity and volume of rectum irradiated are reduced by field shaping and 3-dimensional planning, permitting the administration of higher radiation doses.

Hormone therapy May be given as the sole local treatment for patients not deemed suitable for surgery or radiotherapy. Alternatively, it may be given as an adjunct to other local treatment with the intention of reducing the chance of local recurrence or metastatic disease.

Metastatic disease

Hormone manipulation To reduce circulating testosterone levels—the mainstay of treatment. Current approaches include:

- GRH agonists—shut down the pituitary-gonadal axis
- cyproterone acetate and flutamide—compete with testosterone at the androgen-binding sites.

Surgery Orchidectomy may be carried out as the initial procedure, or after a therapeutic trial of GRH agonists showing the tumour to be hormone responsive.

Palliative radiotherapy Highly effective in the management of bone metastases.

Prognosis

Stage T2/3 60% 5-year survival; 40% 10-year survival.

Well-differentiated tumours 60% 5-year survival

Poorly differentiated tumours 5% 5-year survival.

Sequelae

Radiotherapy Less than 1% develop rectal radiation damage requiring surgery.

Surgery operative complications include reduced potency and impaired urinary control.

Hormone therapy reduced libido, sweats, 'tumour flare' on initiating treatment with a GRH agonist.

CARCINOMA OF THE PENIS

SCC of the penis is a rare tumour comprising < 0.2% of all male cancers. The incidence is increased in Africa and the Far East where the differential diagnosis includes lymphogranuloma venereum. Embarrassment may contribute to a delay in seeking medical attention.

Risk factors

- Slight concordance in the epidemiology with carcinoma of the cervix, indicating possible common aetiological factors.
- More common in uncircumcised men.
- appears associated with poor hygiene.
- may be preceded by a premalignant lesion, e.g. Bowen's disease, erythroplasia of Queyrat, leukoplakia or Paget's disease.

Staging (→ Table 4.9)

TABLE 4.9 Carcinoma of penis: staging

Tis	Carcinoma in situ
Ta	Noninvasive verrucous carcinoma
T1	Invades subepithelial connective tissue
T2	Invades corpus spongiosum or cavernosum
T3	Invades urethra or prostate
T4	Invades other adjacent tissue
N1	Single superficial inguinal lymph node
N2	Multiple or bilateral superficial inguinal lymph nodes
N3	Deep inguinal or pelvic lymph nodes

Making the diagnosis
Signs and symptoms • Long history of skin irritation progression to
ulceration • Development of inguinal adenopathy • Urethral strictures due
to tumour—very unusual • Erythematous plaque or discrete ulcer apparent
on the inner surface of the prepuce or on the glans • In very advanced
disease much of the penis is destroyed and inguinal adenopathy is common.

Investigations • Biopsy of the primary • FNA of suspicious inguinal
lymph nodes.

Treatment

Early lesions
Surgery Local excision followed by radiotherapy to reduce likelihood of local
recurrence where adequate excision margins have not been obtained.

Radiotherapy On its own produces very good results, particularly when the
lesion encroaches on to the shaft.

Advanced disease
Amputation combined with block dissection of the inguinal nodes.

Metastatic disease
Rarely, chemotherapy may be considered for a patient with a good
performance status.

Prognosis
5-year survival in Stage T1/2:80%; in Stage T3/N1: 50%; with unresectable
lymph nodes: < 10%.

TESTICULAR GERM CELL TUMOURS

These tumours constitute the most common malignancy in men 20–40 years
of age. There are approximately 1400 new cases each year in the UK and the
incidence is rising. The types of tumours are summarized in Table 4.10

Risk factors
- Cryptorchidism.
- Testicular maldescent.
- Infertility.
- Klinefelter's syndrome.
- Age
    — > 50 years for spermatocytic variety of seminoma
    — peak incidence in 20s for malignant teratoma
    — peak incidence in the 30s for seminoma.

TABLE 4.10 Testicular germ cell tumours	
Seminoma	Lymphatic spread to para-aortic nodes; haematogenous spread uncommon, primarily to the lungs; subtypes show a similar pattern of the disease
Mixed seminoma/teratoma	Behaviour tends to be determined by the teratomatous elements; treated as teratoma
Teratoma	Teratoma differentiated are more indolent, with less propensity for metastatic spread. Teratoma undifferentiated and teratoma trophoblastic more aggressive; metastasize readily
Extragonadal teratoma	Rare, characteristically arising in the mediastinum or retroperitoneum; may be associated with high serum markers, bulky disease; poor prognosis

Staging (→ Table 4.11)

TABLE 4.11 Testicular germ cell tumours: staging

Royal Marsden system

I	Confined to the testicle	IV	Extralymphatic metastases
II	Abdominal lymphadenopathy	L1	< 3 lung metastases
A	< 2cm	L2	> 3 lung metastases, < 2 cm
B	2–5 cm	L3	> 3 lung metastases, 1 or more > 2 cm
C	> 5 cm	H+	Liver involvement
III	Supradiaphragmatic lymphadenopathy		
0	No abdominal nodes		
A,B,C	As for stage II		

Making the diagnosis

Signs and symptoms • Unilateral testicular swelling, sometimes associated with pain • More advanced disease—fatigue, weight loss, respiratory symptoms in patients with lung involvement • Unexplained back pain may herald retroperitoneal adenopathy • May be palpable supraclavicular adenopathy • SVCO in teratoma patients with advanced mediastinal disease • Headache from intracerebral metastases • Gynaecomastia resulting from tumour production of HCG occasionally seen.

Investigations • Testicular ultrasound • Serum AFP from yolk sac elements—not present in seminomas • HCG—secreted by syncytiotrophoblastic cells • Human placental lactogen—seminomas • Lactate dehydrogenase—often raised in metastatic disease • CXR • CT scan—thorax, abdomen, pelvis • Fundoscopy—may reveal papilloedema • Brain (CT/MR) scan—when cerebral metastases suspected.

Histology
- Seminoma Major histological subtypes include classical, lymphocytic, syncytiotrophoblastic.
- Teratoma.
- Mixed seminoma/teratoma.

The two histological classifications in current usage are the British Testicular Tumour Panel and the World Health Organization (WHO) system (Table 4.12).

TABLE 4.12 Testicular germ cell tumours: classifications

British Testicular Tumour Panel	WHO
Seminoma	Seminoma
Teratoma differentiated (TD)	Teratoma
Malignant teratoma intermediate (MTI)	—mature
Malignant teratoma undifferentiated (MTU)	—immature
Malignant teratoma trophoblastic (MTT)	Teratoma with malignant transformation
Yolk sac tumour	Embryonal carcinoma and teratoma
	Embryonal carcinoma
	Polyembryoma
	Choriocarcinoma ± embryonal carcinoma teratoma
	Yolk sac tumour

Treatment
Surgery Inguinal orchidectomy. Avoid transscrotal orchidectomy as this disrupts normal lymphatic drainage and may lead to scrotal seeding of tumour and inguinal node involvement.

Postoperative management—seminoma
Stage I
- Postorchidectomy radiotherapy to the para-aortic nodes and ipsilateral pelvic nodes.
- Surveillance policy—requires intensive follow-up policy with regular CT scanning to detect and treat early relapse.
- Low-dose radiation confined to the para-aortic region. This approach is relatively free of toxicity.

Stage II A,B
- Abdominal radiotherapy.

Stage II CV Chemotherapy alternatives:
- combination chemotherapy with cisplatin (see below)
- single-agent carboplatin.

Post-operative management—teratoma
Stage I

- Postorchidectomy surveillance policy is generally accepted practice in the UK with monthly follow-up for first year, becoming progressively less frequent thereafter, to include physical examination, CXR, serum AFP and HCG estimations.
- Identification of poor-prognosis Stage I patients with relapse rate of up to 50% consider postsurgery chemotherapy.

Recurrent disease

Approximately 20–25% relapse rate, mostly within first 12 months of follow-up.

- Chemotherapy—effects a cure in most cases.
- Retroperitoneal lymph node dissection (RPLND)—used for these cases in a number of centres outside the UK.

Metastatic teratoma All patients receive chemotherapy, with platinum-containing regimens the mainstay. Drugs commonly used in combination with cisplatin or carboplatin include: • etoposide • vinblastine • bleomycin • ifosfamide • methotrexate.

Treatment usually continues for 4–6 cycles, depending upon response (commonly 2 cycles beyond marker remission). More intensive chemotherapy regimens—incorporating haemopoietic growth factors (GCSF) and marrow ablative chemotherapy—are being evaluated for very poor-prognosis patients and relapsed cases.

Residual lymph node masses May occur in up to 25% of patients after chemotherapy, representing mature teratoma in most cases. Despite benign morphology, they may harbour viable malignant cells and should be surgically removed.

Prognosis

A poor prognosis is associated with the following features:

- poor pretreatment performance status
- tumour bulk > 10 cm
- extranodal involvement, particularly CNS, liver, lung (L3), bone, GI tract
- markedly elevated HCG > 1×10^4 IU/L and AFP > 1×10^3 IU/L.

Stage I seminoma > 96% disease free following orchidectomy and low-dose radiation to para-aortic region.

'Good risk' metastatic teratoma 75–85% 5-year survival.

'Bad risk' metastatic teratoma 60% 5-year survival.

Stage IIC seminoma 85% 5-year survival.

GYNAECOLOGICAL TUMOURS

CARCINOMA OF THE OVARY

Ovarian carcinoma is the fifth commonest cancer in women (1:70), with a higher proportion in industrialized nations, and is increasing in incidence. Most patients present with advanced disease. The tumour is not definitely prevented by prophylactic oophorectomy (peritoneal tumours may then occur).

Risk factors
- Age—commonest between 60 and 85 years of age.
- More common in nulliparous women.
- Less common in users of the oral contraceptive pill (in proportion to duration of use).
- Associated with an increased risk of breast cancer in families with the Lynch II syndrome.
- Associated with a raised tumour marker CA125 in 80% of cases.

Making the diagnosis

Signs and symptoms
Early ovarian carcinoma Normally asymptomatic.

More advanced disease Presents with: • abdominal pain • distension • weight loss • ascites (common feature) • vaginal bleeding (occasional feature).

Investigations • Abdominal ultrasound • TVU • Serum CA125 (ascites also causes a rise in CA125) • Laparoscopy • Ascitic aspiration—cytology • CT scan • In most cases diagnosis is made at laparotomy.

Staging (→ Table 4.13)

Histology
- Epithelial 85–90%
  — serous cystadenocarcinoma
  — mucinous cystadenocarcinoma
  — endometrioid carcinoma
  — undifferentiated carcinoma
  — clear cell carcinoma.
- Germ cell.
- Granulosa cell.
- Borderline.

TABLE 4.13 FIGO staging (Fédération Internationale Gynécologie Oncologie)

Stage I	Limited to ovaries
a	1 ovary; no ascites; no tumour on external surface; capsule intact
b	Both ovaries; no ascites; no tumour on external surfaces; capsule intact
c	Tumour on ovary surface; or capsule ruptured; or ascites containing malignant cells; or positive peritoneal washings
Stage II	With pelvic extension
a	Extension ± metastases to the uterus and/or tubes
b	Extension to other pelvic tissues
c	IIa or IIb with tumour on ovary surface; or with capsule ruptured; or with ascites containing malignant cells; or with positive peritoneal washings
Stage III	Peritoneal implants outside the pelvis ± positive retroperitoneal or inguinal nodes; superficial liver metastases; histologically proven extension to the pelvic small bowel or omentum
a	Tumour grossly limited to the true pelvis with negative nodes but histologically proven microscopic seeding of abdominal peritoneal surfaces
b	Histologically confirmed implants of abdominal peritoneal surfaces, ≤ 2 cm diameter; nodes negative
c	Abdominal implants > 2 cm diameter ± positive retroperitoneal or inguinal nodes
Stage IV	Distant metastases; cytologically malignant pleural effusion; parenchymal liver metastases

 Women < 20 years are much more likely to have a diagnosis of germ cell tumour. Fertility should be preserved by avoiding radical surgery.

Treatment

Each patient should be staged as accurately as possible (including presence, amount and cytology of ascites) both to enable a decision on the need for adjuvant chemotherapy and to improve the accuracy of prognosis.

Surgery This is the mainstay of treatment. The aim should be to remove (debulk) as much of the tumour as possible by total abdominal hysterectomy (TAH), bilateral salpingo-oophorectomy (BSO) and omentectomy performed through a vertical abdominal incision.

'Second-look' surgery To assess response to chemotherapy—less commonly practised in the UK but may be performed to debulk further disease which has responded well to chemotherapy.

Chemotherapy (Table 4.14)

TABLE 4.14 Carcinoma of the ovary: response to chemotherapy

Duration of response	Response to platinum rechallenge
> 2 years	60%
1–2 years	30%
< 2 years	17%

Stage Ic disease Treatment is currently being investigated, the alternative to chemotherapy being a 'wait and watch' policy.

Stage II–IV disease Response to adjuvant chemotherapy with platinum-based drugs cisplatin or carboplatin given monthly for 6 months is 60%. Response may be measured by CT scan.

- Combination chemotherapy (e.g. cyclophosphamide, adriamycin and cisplatin—CAP) has not been shown to be superior to delivery of adequate doses of single-agent platinum.
- Patients should be given adjuvant chemotherapy to reduce the risk of relapse, even if there is no evidence of residual disease postoperatively.
- In the elderly or frail patient, oral chemotherapy (e.g. chlorambucil or melphalan) is occasionally given with palliative intent.

Radiotherapy Seldom used in palliation or in an adjuvant setting. Abdomino-pelvic irradiation is associated with significant morbidity (diarrhoea, adhesions) and is not recommended as routine treatment of ovarian carcinoma.

Relapsed disease
If elevated CA125 falls with treatment, a subsequent increase may signify relapsed disease with a lead time of approximately 3 months. CT scan may confirm the site(s) of disease: if clinically significant ± causing symptoms, 'second-line' chemotherapy may be appropriate. At relapse, the likelihood of responding to rechallenge with platinum is determined by the duration of response (Table 4.14). Other drugs, e.g. carboplatin, melphalan and more recently taxol, may be given. In unresponsive intra-abdominal disease intestinal obstruction is common and may require surgical intervention (see pp. 31–34). Intra-abdominal relapse is often located under the right hemidiaphragm and is inaccessible to radiotherapy.

Prognosis

Grade of tumour and stage at diagnosis are predictive (Table 4.15). 70% of women present with stage III or IV disease.

TABLE 4.15 Carcinoma of the ovary: prognosis

Stage	5-year survival
Ia,b	72%
Ic	60%
II	45%
III	17%
IV	5%

GERM CELL OVARIAN TUMOURS

Unilateral salpingo-oophorectomy only should be performed with no adjuvant treatment, but 10% of tumours are bilateral so the contralateral ovary should be biopsied. 20% of these patients relapse and at that stage radiotherapy and chemotherapy are recommended because the tumour is curable in 50% of patients. Fertility can be preserved with low-dose radiotherapy and platinum-based chemotherapy.

CARCINOMA OF THE CERVIX

Cervical cancer is the most common female malignancy in the Third World. The incidence (including in situ disease) is 24 per 100 000 in the UK, affecting 3% of all women. The peak age for invasive carcinoma is 50–60 years, and for in situ disease approximately 30–40 years. SCC usually originates from the squamous columnar junction of the endocervical canal.

Risk factors

* Associated with a sexually transmissible agent, e.g. human papilloma virus (type 16).
* Frequently associated with chronic cervicitis and cervical dysplasia.
* 30–40% of patients with untreated cervical intraepithelial neoplasia (CIN) III progress to invasive SCC with a latent period of 10–20 years.
* More common in lower socioeconomic groups.
* Associated with cigarette smoking.

Staging (→ Table 4.16)

CIN are graded from I to III on the degree of cellular atypia.

Table 4.16 Carcinoma of the cervix: FIGO staging	
0	Carcinoma in situ
I	Confined to the cervix
a	Microinvasive
b	Invasive
II	
a	Extension to upper 2/3 of vagina
b	Parametrial involvement—not reaching the pelvic sidewall
III	
a	Extension to lower 1/3 of vagina
b	Involvement of pelvic sidewall or causing hydronephrosis
IV	Involvement of bladder, rectum or spread outside the pelvis

Making the diagnosis

Signs and symptoms • Screening diagnosis from cervical smear (CIN III or invasive carcinoma) • Vaginal bleeding (intermenstrual/postcoital or postmenopausal) • Discharge • At vaginal examination the tumour may be exophytic, ulcerative or infiltrating in nature causing a barrel-shaped enlargement of cervix. *Suggestive of advanced disease*: • Low back pain • Weight loss • Rectal and bladder symptoms

Investigations • Examination under GA for staging purposes • Rectal examination to assess parametrial involvement • Cystoscopy—when bladder involvement is suspected • Histological confirmation of primary tumour • CXR • FBC and biochemistry • Transrectal ultrasound • IVU • Abdominal CT/MR scan.

Histology
- SCC: 85–90%.
- Adenocarcinoma or mixed adenosquamous: 10–15%.

Treatment

Stage 0
- Cone biopsy.
- Laser/cryoablation.
- Hysterectomy—may be recommended in postmenopausal women.

Early stage (I and II)
Radiotherapy and radical surgery are equally effective in terms of local control and overall survival.

Radiotherapy Usually a combination of external beam and intracavitary.
• External beam therapy—encompasses the parametrium and pelvic lymph nodes • Intracavitary treatment—gives a high dose confined to the uterus and upper vagina.

Surgery • Wertheim hysterectomy—more commonly undertaken in young medically fit patients. Occasionally 1 ovary is conserved in premenopausal women • Postoperative radiation—may be offered depending upon histological findings.

Stage III and IV
Radiotherapy The mainstay of treatment, the major component delivered as external beam to the pelvis.

Neoadjuvant chemotherapy Its place is currently under evaluation.

Recurrent disease
Curative treatment The salvage rate is disappointing. • Early-stage disease recurrence following radiotherapy may be amenable to curative surgery if recurrence is localized • Local recurrence following Wertheim hysterectomy may be cured by pelvic radiation.

Palliative treatment In most cases therapy for recurrence is palliative.
• Palliative combination chemotherapy for recurrence in a previously irradiated area or metastatic disease has a response rate of approximately 30–40% • Active drugs include methotrexate, cisplatin, mitomycin C, bleomycin and doxorubicin.

Prognosis
5-year survival for stage I: 85%; Stage II: 55%; Stage III: 35%; Stage IV: 5%.

Sequelae
Radiotherapy-related • Late—rectal, bladder, small bowel damage: onset 6–24 months, < 5% of cases may require surgery • Menopausal symptoms (may be safely treated by HRT) • Dyspareunia can occur following both radiotherapy and surgery.

CARCINOMA OF UTERINE BODY

Uterine cancer occurs predominantly in postmenopausal women. Early presentation leads to a favourable prognosis compared with the other major gynaecological malignancies. The incidence in the UK is 14 per 100 000, with considerable geographic variation.

Risk factors
Associated with: • endometrial hyperplasia • nulliparity • late menopause • obesity • diabetes mellitus • hypertension • high-oestrogen oral contraceptive pill • tamoxifen.

Staging
In 75% of cases the tumour is confined to the uterus at initial diagnosis. The tumour spreads into the endometrium and invades the muscle, the degree of myometrial infiltration being an important prognostic factor. The incidence of nodal involvement increases with FIGO stage (Table 4.17), degree of muscle invasion and histological grade. The vagina is a common site for the seeding of tumour nodules.

TABLE 4.17 Carcinoma of uterus: FIGO clinical staging	
I	Confined to corpus
a	< 8 cm
b	> 8 cm
II	Extension to cervix
III	Beyond the uterus but confined to within the pelvis
IV	
a	Bladder, rectum, outside true pelvis
b	Distant metastases, predominantly in lung and liver

Making the diagnosis
Signs and symptoms
• Vaginal bleeding—presenting symptom in 70–80% of cases
  — postmenopausal bleeding leads to early presentation (only 20% of cases occur in premenopausal women).
• Vaginal discharge—30%.
• Pain and weight loss—associated with advanced disease.
• An enlarged uterus may be palpable per abdomen, but pelvic examination is often uninformative in early-stage disease.

Investigations • D&C for histological confirmation of primary tumour • CXR • FBC and biochemistry.

Histology
- Adenocarcinoma: 80–90%.
- Adeno-acanthoma: 5–10%.
- Leiomyosarcoma: < 5%.

Treatment
Surgery The mainstay of treatment, comprising total abdominal hysterectomy and bilateral salpingo-oophorectomy (TAH and BSO).

Adjuvant therapy Recommended after surgery for patients with the following poor prognostic features: • > 1/3 myometrial infiltration • poorly differentiated carcinomas • lymph node involvement.

Radiotherapy Comprises external beam treatment to the pelvis ± local irradiation to the vaginal vault. Radiotherapy alone is given to patients medically unfit for surgery.

Recurrent disease
In most cases therapy for recurrence is palliative. Medroxyprogesterone acetate is associated with a very low response rate. However, it is non-toxic and may be associated with an enhanced feeling of well-being.

Prognosis
5-year survival with Stage I, 85%; Stage II, 65%; Stage III, 35%; Stage IV, 5%.

Sequelae
As for carcinoma of the cervix.

CARCINOMA OF THE VAGINA

Vaginal cancer counts for 1–2% of gynaecological malignancies. The predominantly SCCs occur mostly in the 50–70 year age group. It may be difficult to distinguish a vaginal primary from secondary deposits from uterus or vulva. Tumours frequently appear on the posterior wall of the upper third of the vagina and can spread along the vaginal wall to invade the cervix and vulva. The absence of anatomical barriers permits unimpeded tumour extension into the rectum or bladder. Inguinal nodes are most commonly affected.

Risk factors
- SCC: associated with long-term use of vaginal ring pessaries.
- Clear cell adenocarcinoma in young women: maternal stilboestrol therapy for threatened abortion (no longer practised).

Staging (→ Table 4.18)

	TABLE 4.18 Carcinoma of vagina: FIGO clinical staging
0	Carcinoma in situ
I	Confined to vaginal mucosa
II	Subvaginal infiltration
a	No parametrial involvement
b	Parametrial involvement
III	Tumour extending to pelvic sidewall
IV	Tumour extension to bladder, rectum, or spread outside pelvis

Making the diagnosis
Signs and symptoms • Blood-stained vaginal discharge—presenting symptom in 50–75% of cases • Urinary, rectal symptoms or pain—indicative of advanced disease • Fistula formation—may occur in advanced cases.

Investigations • Thorough speculum examination • Exfoliative cytology may pick up early lesions—may present as vaginal intraepithelial neoplasia (VAIN) • Palpation reveals extent of infiltration • EUA and biopsy • D&C—may be required to exclude uterine primary • CXR • FBC and biochemistry • CT or MR scan.

Histology
- SCC—most cases.
- Adenocarcinoma—accounts for 5% of vaginal tumours arising from glandular epithelium.
- Other vaginal tumours include soft tissue sarcomas (sarcoma botryoides in children) and malignant melanoma.

Treatment
Surgery As this disease predominantly affects the elderly population, in most cases surgery is inappropriate. • Total vaginectomy, TAH with pelvic lymphadenectomy for early lesions • Pelvic exenteration for distal lesions because of proximity of rectum and bladder.

Radiotherapy • In situ disease can be treated with intravaginal applicator • Invasive disease—treated with external beam therapy.

Recurrent disease
Recurrence following pelvic clearance may be treated by radiotherapy, usually with palliative intent.

Prognosis

5-year survival with Stage I, 75%; Stage II, 55%; Stage III, 25%; Stage IV, < 5%.

Sequelae

- Disease related: haemorrhage, sepsis, proctitis, cystitis, fistulae.
- Treatment related: dyspareunia, proctitis, cystitis, fistulae.

CARCINOMA OF THE VULVA

Carcinoma of the vulva comprises 4% of gynaecological malignancy. It is rare before the age of 50, and concealment in an elderly population often gives rise to advanced disease at presentation.

Over 70% of cases arise in the labia majora and labia minora, and tumours may spread to the vagina, urethra and perineum. The inguinal lymph nodes are the first to be involved, and are present in up to 50% of patients at presentation. Approximately 20% of patients with histologically proven inguinal node disease will also have pelvic node involvement.

Risk factors

- Aetiological factors include leukoplakia and other chronic vulval dystrophies.
- Associated with diabetes mellitus.

Staging (→ Table 4.19)

TABLE 4.19 Carcinoma of vulva: staging	
T1	Confined to vulva, < 2 cm
T2	Confined to vulva, > 2 cm
T3	Spread to urethra, vagina, perineum
T4	
a	Spread to bladder
b	Spread to rectum, outside pelvis
Stage I	No palpable nodes
Stage II	No palpable nodes
Stage III	No palpable nodes
Stage IV	Fixed nodes

Making the diagnosis

Signs and symptoms • Pruritus vulvae • Ulceration • Discharge • Fissuring • Asymptomatic primary, but presenting with inguinal lymph node enlargement • Vulval mass or evidence of extensive field change over the vulva.

Investigations • Physical examination to exclude secondary deposits from endometrium, cervix, large bowel • Biopsy and histological confirmation • FNAC of nodes • CXR • FBC and biochemistry • CT scan for pelvic nodal assessment. In view of frequent inflammatory inguinal adenopathy, clinical lymph node assessment may be inaccurate.

Differential diagnosis
Primary chronic vulvitis, vulval condylomata, lymphogranuloma inguinale and venereum.

Secondary endometrium, cervix, large bowel.

Histology
- SCC: > 90%. May be associated with multifocal areas of carcinoma in situ.
- Other vulval tumours: < 10%. Paget's disease, adenocarcinoma (arising in Bartholin's gland), malignant melanoma, basal cell carcinoma, adenoid cystic carcinoma.

Treatment
Surgery Careful follow-up of premalignant lesions is important. • Wide local excision may be adequate for a focus of preinvasive disease • Simple vulvectomy appropriate for local lesion • Radical vulvectomy with unilateral or bilateral block nodal dissection for more advanced lesions.

Radiotherapy The vulva does not tolerate radiotherapy well. • Interstitial irradiation in posterior lesions where surgery may jeopardize the anal sphincter • Palliative external beam therapy is rarely effective.

Recurrent disease
Recurrence following radical surgery is invariably incurable. Management is symptomatic.

Prognosis
Related to staging (Table 4.20).

TABLE 4.20 Carcinoma of the vulva: prognosis	
Stage	**5-year survival**
Resectable, no nodes	75%
Resectable, inguinal and femoral nodes	25%
Resectable, pelvic nodes	< 20%

TUMOURS OF THE HEAD AND NECK

CARCINOMA OF THE LIP

Carcinoma of the lip usually presents early and consequently carries a good prognosis. It arises from vermilion border. The lower lip is most commonly affected (95%). There is a male predominance of > 10:1.

Risk factors
Associated with • sun damage and • leukoplakia.

Staging (→ Table 4.21)

TABLE 4.21 Carcinoma of the lip: Staging

T1	< 2 cm
T2	2–4 cm
T3	> 4 cm
T4	Invasion beyond lip (tongue, bone, floor of mouth)
N1	Ipsilateral lymph node < 3cm in diameter
N2	
a	Single ipsilateral lymph node 3–6 cm in diameter
b	Multiple ipsilateral lymph nodes < 6cm
c	Bilateral or contralateral lymph nodes < 6 cm
N3	Lymph node > 6 cm in diameter

Making the diagnosis
• Lesion is easily apparent.
• Initial differential diagnosis includes infective and traumatic origin.
• Histological confirmation is essential.
• In the absence of clinical evidence of advanced disease no further investigations routinely required.
• < 10% of patients have nodal disease at presentation.

Histology
Predominantly SCC, with adenoid cystic carcinoma on the inner surface of the lip.

Treatment
Overall, the results from surgery and radiotherapy are comparable in terms of local control and cosmesis.

Surgery • Wide local excision • Block dissection if nodal involvement.

Radiotherapy Interstitial or external beam therapy to primary tumour.

CARCINOMA OF THE ORAL CAVITY

Carcinoma of the oral cavity comprises 2% of malignant tumours in the UK and may occur at the following sites: tongue (ant 2/3, 35%), floor of mouth (25%), buccal mucosa (15%), lower alveolus (15%), upper alveolus (5%), hard palate (5%).

Risk factors
• Poor dental hygiene, alcohol, smoking.
• Betel nut chewing, e.g. in India.
• Areas of unstable epithelium within the oral cavity—may give rise to multiple tumours.
• Leukoplakia—may precede invasive carcinoma.

Staging (→ Table 14.22)

TABLE 4.22 Carcinoma of the oral cavity: staging	
The incidence of nodal disease correlates with size of the primary tumour. N0 frequency: T1 95%, T2 85%, T3 50%.	
T1	< 2 cm
T2	2–4 cm
T3	> 4 cm
T4	Invasion into adjacent structures
N1	Ipsilateral lymph node < 3 cm
N2	
a	Single ipsilateral lymph node 3–6 cm
b	Multiple ipsilateral lymph nodes < 6 cm
c	Bilateral or contralateral lymph nodes < 6 cm
N3	Lymph node > 6 cm

Making the diagnosis
• Small ulcer—often attributed to abrasion on a rough tooth or ill-fitting dentures.
• Node involvement in approximately 25% of patients.
• Nodal disease—occurs largely in the submandibular, submental and upper deep cervical lymph nodes.

Investigations
- Thorough examination of the oral cavity, including
  — accurate assessment of the site and extent of the primary tumour
  — evaluation of dental health and nodal status.
- CXR
  — a second bronchogenic primary in a heavy cigarette smoker
  — pulmonary secondaries (more common in adenoid cystic carcinoma).
- Orthopantomogram (OPG) if tumour approximates to mandible.
- CT/MR scan
  — may define tumour extent more clearly, e.g. adenoid cystic carcinoma
  — provides more accurate nodal assessment.

Histology
SCC 95% (often well differentiated).

Adenoid cystic < 5% (i.e. hard palate).

Treatment

Primary tumour
Local control of most early-stage tumours is equivalent with surgery or radiotherapy. Treatment depends upon patient fitness for surgery and the acute and late morbidity of the two approaches.

Advanced disease
- Surgery followed by radiotherapy to reduce the chance of subsequent recurrence.
- Primary radiotherapy by external beam treatment or interstitial therapy, followed by elective surgical excision or salvage surgery on recurrence— interstitial treatment is performed on small (T1, T2) tumours, e.g. lateral border of the tongue, using caesium needles or iridium wire to limit volume of normal tissue irradiated, thus reducing morbidity.

Lymph nodes
N0 disease
- Adjuvant treatment—tends to be given to patients at high risk of nodal recurrence:
  1. surgery (block dissection)
  2. lymph node irradiation
- 'Watch' policy with salvage neck dissection following nodal recurrence— for low risk patients.

Clinically involved neck nodes
- Surgery to primary and neck dissection.
- Radiotherapy to primary and neck dissection.
- Radiotherapy to primary and nodal areas with surgery on relapse.

These treatment choices require careful collaboration between surgeon and clinical oncologist.

Chemotherapy • Regimens include methotrexate, cisplatin, 5FU bleomycin and vinblastine • Response rates approximately 30–40% • The place of adjuvant chemotherapy has not yet been proven.

Palliation

Radiotherapy May offer worthwhile palliation when patients present with advanced incurable disease.

Chemotherapy In advanced or recurrent disease can bring about effective palliation.

Prognosis

At T1 stage, 90% primary tumour control; all failures should be salvaged. At T2, 75% primary tumour control; 50% of failures are salvaged. At T3, 50% primary tumour control; few salvaged.

Sequelae

Radiotherapy-related
- Acute—painful mucosa, impeding dietary intake.
  — adequate analgesia
  — appropriate nutritional support during the treatment and for several weeks afterwards.
- Late
  — altered taste in the irradiated area
  — reduced salivary output
  — accelerated tooth decay
  — osteoradionecrosis in < 5% of cases treated with radical radiotherapy— more commonly seen in the mandible, particularly following tooth extraction.

Disease-related
Second malignancy—within oral cavity in 6% of patients.

- Nutritional support is very important during and shortly after treatment until mucositis resolves.
- Education is required regarding oro-dental hygiene.
- Patients *must* stop smoking.
- In view of the similar risk factors, there is an increased incidence of a subsequent bronchogenic primary.

CARCINOMA OF THE OROPHARYNX

SCC of the oropharynx has an incidence of 1:100 000 in the UK, with a slight male predominance (1.6:1). Non-Hodgkin's lymphoma may arise in Waldeyer's ring. SCC of the oropharynx has a propensity for early nodal spread, initially to the jugulodigastric region.

Risk factors
Poor dental hygiene, alcohol, smoking.

Staging (→ Table 4.23)

TABLE 4.23 Carcinoma of the oropharynx: staging	
T1	< 2 cm
T2	2–4 cm
T3	> 4 cm
T4	Invasion beyond tonsil (tongue, bone, floor of mouth)
N1	Ipsilateral lymph node < 3 cm
N2	
a	Single ipsilateral lymph node 3–6 cm
b	Multiple ipsilateral lymph nodes < 6 cm
c	Bilateral or contralateral lymph nodes < 6 cm
N3	Lymph node > 6 cm

Making the diagnosis
Signs and symptoms • Discomfort in the throat, occasionally associated with the sensation of a foreign body • Otalgia—indicative of advanced disease • Dysphagia and weight loss—indicative of advanced disease • May present as a node in the neck, requiring a thorough examination of the oropharynx.

Investigations • Accurate assessment of the site and extent of the primary tumour • Careful palpation of the neck for nodal disease • Biopsy at EUA for histological confirmation • CXR.

Treatment
Similar approach to oral cavity.

Surgery Less commonly undertaken in the UK.

Adjuvant treatment of nodal areas Recommended for tumours beyond T1 either using neck irradiation or block dissection of the neck.

CARCINOMA OF THE NASOPHARYNX

SCC of the nasopharynx is a rare tumour in the UK but common in the Far East. The tumour usually originates either on the roof or in the fossa of Rosenmuller and spreads posterolaterally to the parapharyngeal space involving the last 4 cranial nerves and mandibular branch of the trigeminal as it emerges from the foramen ovale. The trigeminal and facial nerves may be involved directly by invasion through the foramen lacerum. Direct spread also occurs inferiorly into oropharynx, superiorly through the skull base laterally to involve the eustachian tube and anteriorly into the nasal cavity.

Risk factors
* Epstein–Barr viral infection in Far East.
* Salted fish.
* Vitamin C deficiency.

Staging (→ Table 4.24)

TABLE 4.24 Carcinoma of nasopharynx: staging

T1	1 subsite*
T2	2 subsites
T3	Into nasal cavity or oropharynx
T4	Bone erosion or cranial nerve involvement

*Subsites: *1* posterosuperior aspect; *2* lateral wall; *3* inferior aspect

Making the diagnosis
Signs and symptoms • Frequently presents late, with enlarged cervical lymph nodes • Early lymph node involvement, including retropharyngeal and cervical nodes • Downward displacement of the soft palate may be visible within the oral cavity • Nasal obstruction • Pain (mandibular division of trigeminal) • Otalgia • Dysphagia • Cranial nerve palsies • Hearing loss • Epistaxis • Evidence of disseminated lymphadenopathy on further examination suggests a diagnosis of non-Hodgkin's lymphoma.

Investigations • EUA to investigate primary tumour • Examination of cranial nerves • Careful palpation of the neck • Multiple biopsies, including blind biopsies of the nasopharynx in 'neck node only' presentations • CXR • X-rays of the postnasal space and base of skull • CT or MR scan.

Histology
* SCC most common.
* Other tumour types: non-Hodgkin's lymphoma, adenocarcinoma, malignant melanoma.

Treatment
Surgery Rarely possible.

Radiotherapy The treatment of choice for the primary tumour. Adjuvant radiotherapy to the regional nodal areas should be carried out in all cases.

Young patients
Combination treatment with chemotherapy and irradiation for chemosensitive EBV-associated nasopharyngeal carcinoma and tumours.

Prognosis
T1 60% 5-year survival

Overall 30–35% 5-year survival as most patients present with advanced disease

Sequelae
Similar to carcinoma of the oral cavity.

CARCINOMA OF THE HYPOPHARYNX

SCC of the hypopharynx occurs with an incidence of 1 per 100 000 in the UK. It may arise in the pyriform sinus, the posterior pharyngeal wall or the postcricoid region. With the exception of postcricoid carcinoma it is more common in men than women. Local spread occurs by submucosal infiltration to involve the larynx and thyroid cartilage and inferiorly to the upper oesophagus. Blood-borne metastases are rare.

Risk factors
- Postcricoid carcinoma associated with pharyngeal web and iron deficiency anaemia (Paterson–Kelly syndrome) in women.
- Incidence of SCC in other sites associated with cigarette smoking and alcohol intake.

Staging (→ Table 4.25)

TABLE 4.25 Carcinoma of hypopharynx: staging	
T1	1 subsite*
T2	> 1 subsite, or adjacent site—no fixation of hemilarynx
T3	> 1 subsite, or adjacent site—fixation of hemilarynx
T4	Invades an adjacent structure

*Subsites: *1* postcricoid; *2* pyriform sinus; *3* posterior pharyngeal wall

Making the diagnosis

Signs and symptoms • Foreign body sensation in the throat—late presentation • Cervical lymphadenopathy—late presentation • Dysphagia: appears relatively early in postcricoid carcinoma and develops late in posterior pharyngeal wall lesions • Pain and weight loss—indicative of advanced disease • Cervical node involvement—common at presentation and frequently bilateral.

Investigations • Asessment of general health is important indicator of disease progression and is a guide to suitability for radical surgery or radiotherapy • Indirect or direct laryngoscopy to assess local tumour extent • Palpation of the neck will indicate the presence of nodal disease • EUA and biopsy • X-rays: soft tissue lateral films of neck reveal widening of the prevertebral space; barium swallow (postcricoid); chest • CT/MR scan.

Treatment

Surgery Laryngopharyngectomy with radical neck dissection. In view of late presentation, the disease may be beyond curative resection.

Radiotherapy May be given as initial treatment with surgery on relapse. However, follow-up assessment of hypopharynx is difficult, and the recurrent disease may be too advanced or the patient too frail for salvage surgery.

Chemotherapy As adjuvant therapy its role has not yet been confirmed. Chemotherapy palliation of recurrent or metastatic disease with current agents is disappointing.

Prognosis

Survival by stage is similar to oral cavity. Overall: 20–30% 5-year survival.

Sequelae

Strictures may develop several months post radiotherapy due to fibrotic changes and may require dilatation.

CARCINOMA OF THE LARYNX

SCC of the larynx comprises 2% of malignant tumours in the UK with an incidence of 4:100 000. There is a male preponderance (7:1) and geographical variation, being more common in parts of South America and India. Local spread is slow and nodal disease uncommon. Supraglottic carcinoma presents with more advanced local disease. Subglottic carcinoma is rare and lymphatic spread to paratracheal nodes occurs readily.

• Glottic—vocal cords joined by anterior and posterior commissures; usually presents early.

- Supraglottic—from inferior surface of epiglottis to vocal cords; usually presents with more advanced local disease.
- Subglottic—from vocal cords to opening of the trachea at the inferior border of the cricoid cartilage; rare.

Risk factors
Associated with tobacco smoking.

Staging (→ Table 4.26)

TABLE 4.26 Carcinoma of larynx: staging	
Supraglottis	
T1	Confined to 1 subsite* of supraglottis—normal cord mobility
T2	> 1 subsite of supraglottis or glottis—normal cord mobility
T3	Confined to larynx with impaired cord mobility, or spread to postcricoid area, medial wall of pyriform sinus or pre-epiglottic tissues
T4	Invasion into thyroid cartilage ± other tissues beyond the larynx, i.e. oropharynx, soft tissues of the neck
Glottis	
T1	Confined to cords
a	1 cord
b	Both cords
T2	Spread off the cord ± impaired vocal cord mobility
T3	Tumour limited to larynx with fixed cord
T4	Invasion into thyroid cartilage ± other tissues beyond the larynx, i.e. oropharynx, soft tissues of the neck
Subglottis	
T1	Tumour limited to subglottis
T2	Spread to the cord with normal or impaired vocal cord mobility
T3	Tumour limited to larynx with fixed cord
T4	Invasion into thyroid cartilage ± other tissues beyond the larynx, i.e. oropharynx, soft tissues of the neck
*Subsites: 1 epilarynx; 2 supraglottis excluding epilarynx	

Making the diagnosis
Signs and symptoms Usually presents early, sometimes as in situ disease.
- Hoarse voice caused by a small nodule on the vocal cords. *Later features*:
- Stridor in supraglottic tumours • Dysphagia—indicates pharyngeal involvement • Otalgia—suggests locally advanced disease • Palpable nodes at presentation—approximately 30% • Cervical nodes at histology 60–70%.

Investigations • Indirect or direct fibreoptic laryngoscopy to assess tumour extent • Palpation of the neck—may reveal expansion of larynx, loss of laryngeal crepitus, lymphadenopathy • EUA and biopsy • X-ray—soft-tissue lateral films of neck, laryngeal tomography, chest • CT/MR scan.

Treatment

Early glottic carcinoma
Comparable results with surgery (laryngectomy or cordectomy) and radiotherapy. Stripping of the cords may be adequate for pre-invasive disease, but careful follow-up is necessary.

Surgery Indicated in supra- and subglottic tumours associated with airway obstruction. Nodal disease is treated by block dissection of the neck.

Radiotherapy Allows preservation of the larynx; careful follow-up policy with salvage surgery for recurrent disease. Postoperative radiotherapy should encompass the tracheostomy stoma in order to avoid stomal recurrence.

Prognosis (→ Table 4.27)

TABLE 4.27 Carcinoma of larynx: prognosis	
Stage	5-year survival
Glottis	
I	90%
2	80%
3	55%
4	10%
Supraglottis/subglottis	
Overall	40%

Recurrence
Most common in the first 1–2 years, requiring careful follow-up. Thereafter, outpatient visits can become less frequent. Primary tumour recurrence is very rare beyond 5 years.

Sequelae
Treatment-related • Surgery—postlaryngectomy speech therapy
• Radiotherapy—acute mucosal reaction requiring adequate analgesia and nutritional support if necessary; late radiation problems in up to 3% of patients (may require laryngectomy)—more common in patients who continue to smoke.

Disease-related • Second malignancy in the head and neck region
• 5–10% incidence subsequent bronchial primary carcinoma.

CARCINOMA OF THE PARANASAL SINUSES

Paranasal sinus tumours are uncommon. The paranasal sinuses comprise the nasal cavity, maxillary sinus and ethmoid sinus. Tumours are usually squamous cell and are rare < 40 years. Most disease is advanced at the time of presentation and involves several sinuses, making identification of the original site difficult. Nodal involvement occurs late.

Risk factors
• Adenocarcinoma is associated with working with hard woods in the furniture trade.

Making the diagnosis
• Tends to present after spread beyond the sinus.
• Tumour extension occurs superiorly into the anterior and middle cranial fossae, laterally into the orbit or cheek, and inferiorly into the oral cavity.
• Swelling over maxillary antrum or inner canthus.
• Late symptoms include
  — nasal obstruction
  — discharge and epistaxis
  — sinus pain
  — sensation of fullness over the maxilla
  — diplopia and visual disturbance with orbital involvement
  — painful or loose teeth, or ill fitting upper dentures with inferior extension
  — headache, cranial nerve palsies and trismus with posterior tumour spread
  — proptosis or cranial nerve palsies.

Treatment
A combination of radiotherapy and surgery has been advocated as the treatment of choice, but there are no satisfactory comparative studies to confirm this. Cases which are too advanced, or the patient too frail for surgery, are treated by radiation alone.

Surgery Maxillectomy/ethmoidectomy, with orbital exenteration if the orbital wall has been breached.

Radiotherapy The field includes the maxillary antrum, ethmoids and nasal fossa. If there is involvement of the orbit the eye must be included within the treatment field.

Prognosis
Overall: 30–40% 5-year survival.

Sequelae
- Surgery — following maxillectomy a removable obturator facilitates speech and eating and permits direct visualization during follow-up; following orbital exenteration a prosthetic eye is required.
- Radiotherapy — loss of vision in irradiated eye occurs 9–18 months post treatment.

 A lesion on hard palate or upper alveolus—always think of antral tumours.

CARCINOMA OF THE THYROID

Thyroid cancer is relatively uncommon in the UK (1:100 000). Higher incidence has been reported in other countries (e.g. Israel and Iceland—15:100 000). It is more common in women and can occur in early adult life. Papillary carcinoma may be multifocal, with the tumours confined by a false capsule for prolonged periods of time. Lymphatic spread is to the cervical nodes, and distant metastases most commonly to lung. Follicular carcinoma spreads predominantly to lung and bone. Anaplastic carcinoma is seen in the older age group, and runs a more aggressive course with rapid local growth and early lymph node involvement.

Risk factors
Follicular carcinoma • Associated with iodine deficiency.

Papillary carcinoma • Associated with iodine-rich diet • Ionizing radiation—latent period of 10–40 years following exposure to low doses to the neck in childhood (e.g. atomic bomb survivors) • No increased risk observed for radioiodine for thyrotoxicosis • Marginal effect of neck irradiation in Hodgkin's disease.

Medullary carcinoma • Sporadic (80%) • Inherited as a autosomal dominant trait as part of the multiple endocrine neoplasia complex (MEN II or III).

Staging (→ Table 4.28)

TABLE 4.28 Carcinoma of thyroid: staging	
T1	< 1 cm and confined to the thyroid
T2	1–4 cm and confined to the thyroid
T3	> 4 cm and confined to the thyroid
T4	Extension beyond the thyroid capsule

Making the diagnosis

Signs and symptoms • Swelling in the neck of variable duration • Rapidly enlarging thyroid swelling associated with symptoms of compression including hoarse voice, dysphagia or stridor suggests advanced disease • Most patients are clinically euthyroid.

Investigations • IDL if there is hoarseness • Radionuclide thyroid imaging (suspicious 'cold' nodule) • Ultrasound (thyroid cysts) • X-ray chest, thoracic inlet, barium swallow • CT/MR scan (if locally advanced) • FNAC (cysts or anaplastic carcinoma) — difficult to interpret if well-differentiated carcinoma is suspected • Thyroid function tests and thyroid antibodies (exclude Hashimoto's disease).

Treatment

Surgery The suspicious solitary nodule should be removed by total lobectomy, to avoid re-operating on that side if cancer is diagnosed. Following diagnosis, total thyroidectomy, sparing recurrent laryngeal nerves and parathyroids, should ideally be undertaken. Adjacent involved lymph nodes are removed, but a full block dissection is not mandatory.

For anaplastic carcinoma, an isthmusectomy may be preferable to relieve stridor (see pp. 23–24).

Radiotherapy

Papillary and follicular carcinoma The amount of residual thyroid tissue post surgery is assessed by radionuclide imaging, and thyroid remnant is ablated with ^{131}Iodine.

Metastatic disease Isotope screening 3 months post ablation.

Bulky residual tumour or when thyroid ablation is inadequate External beam therapy to the thyroid and upper mediastinum.

Recurrent disease

Repeated surgery For subsequent local or nodal recurrence of papillary carcinoma—offers an excellent prospect of cure.

Chemotherapy Achieves response rates of the order of 20–30% in metastatic or recurrent disease.

Prognosis (→Table 4.29)

TABLE 4.29 Comparative incidence and survival rates for thyroid cancers

Histology	% incidence	Survival
Papillary carcinoma	60	> 95% at 15 years
Follicular carcinoma	20	
non-invasive		86% at 10 years
angioinvasive		50–60% at 10 years
Anaplastic carcinoma	15	< 5% at 5 years
Medullary carcinoma	5	65% at 10 years
Non-Hodgkin's lymphoma	1	
Soft-tissue sarcoma	1	

Sequelae

Thyroxine replacement Following thyroid ablation the TSH level must remain suppressed, and therefore patients are maintained on adequate doses of thyroxine replacement.

Treatment-related • Surgery — immediate hypocalcaemia due to interference with parathyroids • Radiotherapy — post high-dose thyroid ablation: fatigue, anorexia, short-lived swelling of the neck and transient bone marrow suppression.

 Men should be advised not to father children for at least 3 months, and women should not become pregnant within 6 months of ^{131}I ablation therapy.

TUMOURS OF THE SALIVARY GLANDS

These tumours can affect any of the major glands (parotid, submandibular and sublingual) and the minor (tiny glands on the palate, lips and buccal mucosa), their incidence tending to reflect the comparative volume of salivary tissue at the different sites, i.e. the parotid gland is the commonest site for these lesions. Warthin's tumour, a benign condition affecting only the parotid gland (sometimes inappropriately known as 'adenolymphoma') has a tendency to recur locally if not adequately excised. The salivary glands are also a common site of involvement by lymphomas (see pp. 150–155).

Histology
- Pleomorphic adenoma (75%).
- Adenocarcinoma (12%).
- Monomorphic adenoma (8%).
- Muco-epidermoid carcinoma, acinic cell carcinoma, adenoid-cystic carcinoma (rare).

PLEOMORPHIC ADENOMA
- Connective tissue stroma contains a mixture of tissue types with cartilagenous and mucous elements predominant (also referred to as a 'mixed parotid tumour').
- Slow growing.
- If left untreated, they tend to grow to a large size which may make nerve-sparing surgery more difficult.
- Occasionally malignant change has been reported—referred to as 'carcinoma ex-pleomorphic adenoma'.

Making the diagnosis
- Difficult to diagnose preoperatively—surgery is often necessary in order to differentiate it from malignant parotid lesions.
- Characterized by lobulated edge.
- Recurrent pleomorphic adenomas are often multifocal.

Treatment
Surgery The tumour is surrounded by an incomplete capsule of compressed parotid and fibrous tissue ('pseudo capsule') which results in a very high incidence of local recurrence if the tumour is simply 'shelled out'.

- Superficial parotidectomy — treatment of choice which maximizes the margin of normal tissue removed around the tumour edge.
- Careful dissection in the extracapsular plane which avoids tumour spillage by taking a small margin of normal tissue.

Recurrent disease
Total parotidectomy (sparing the facial nerve) is usually required, combined with postoperative radiotherapy to the parotid bed to minimize the risk of further recurrence. The risk of nerve damage increases with each subsequent operation.

CARCINOMA OF THE PAROTID

Making the diagnosis
- Rapidly enlarging mass.
- Progressive facial palsy.
- parotid carcinoma (particularly the adenoid-cystic variety) has a propensity for perineural spread towards the skull base.
- FNAC or TruCut biopsy.
- CT scan to outline the extent of disease.

Treatment
Surgery For resectable disease.
- Total parotidectomy, including resection of the facial nerve
  — cable nerve graft (the great auricular nerve) in facial nerve division, as some nerve function may return
  — lateral tarsoraphy and operation to lift the corner of the mouth is often performed simultaneously to minimize the facial nerve defect.
- Radical neck dissection where there is secondary involvement of cervical lymph nodes.

Postoperative radiotherapy To prevent uncontrolled local recurrence at skull base.

Prognosis
Parotid carcinoma tends to present late and therefore carries a poor prognosis.

SKIN TUMOURS

MELANOMA

Cutaneous melanoma is the third commonest skin cancer. The doubling in incidence every 6–10 years may be related to a rise in recreational exposure to sunlight (ultraviolet; UV) and reduction of ozone layer. Rarely, it may regress spontaneously and re-present with metastatic disease.

Risk factors
- Aetiology—UV stimulation of melanocytes at the base of the epidermis.
- Race—cutaneous melanoma affects Caucasians almost exclusively. Highest risk:
  — children with multiple episodes of sunburn
  — people with fair colouring and freckles
  — red hair triples the relative risk
  — acral lentiginous more common in Afro-Caribbean people.
- Age
  — cutaneous melanoma affects younger people (median age 45 years)
  — acral lentiginous more common in people > 60 years.
- Familial in the dysplastic naevus syndrome.
- More common in people who have already had one melanoma resected.

Staging
- Microstaging uses 2 systems
  — Breslow: total vertical height measured from granular layer to the site of deepest penetration
  — Clark: depth of invasion into dermal layers of subcutaneous fat measured (levels II–V).
- Macrostaging is less detailed, considering whether the melanoma
  — is localized (*I*, 85% of cases)
  — has regional metastases (*II*)
  — has distant metastases (*III*).

American Joint Committee on Cancer (AJCC) subdivisions	
IA	Localized melanoma < 0.75 mm or level II (T1N0M0)
IB	Localized melanoma 0.76–1.5 mm or level III (T2N0M0)
IIA	Localized melanoma 1.5–4 mm or level IV (T3N0M0)
IIB	Localized melanoma 4 mm or level V (T4N0M0)
III	Limited nodal metastases involving only 1 regional lymph node basin, or < 5 in transit metastases but without nodal metastases (any T, N1M0)
IV	Advanced regional metastases (any T, N2M0) or any patient with distant metastases (any T, any N, M1 or M2)

Making the diagnosis
- Sudden appearance of a mole or freckle.
- In a pre-existing mole
    — itch
    — bleeding
    — change in colour
    — alteration in shape.
- Melanoma may be amelanotic or depigmented (10% of cases).
- Common sites
    — leg in women
    — trunk in men.

Any such lesion must be excised completely and sent for histological evaluation to exclude malignant melanoma.

Histology (→ Table 4.30)

TABLE 4.30 Melanoma: histology	
Cutaneous melanoma	**90%**
Subtypes	
Superficial spreading	70%; generally arise in pre-existing mole
Nodular	15–30%; more aggressive and usually appear in middle age, especially in men
Lentigo maligna	4–10%; uncommon < 50 years; more common in women; less malignant than the others
Acral lentiginous	More commonly on palms, soles, nails

Treatment

Surgery
Stage I–III (AJCC) Surgical excision — margin depends on thickness and histological type. 1–2 cm minimum margin, rising to 3 cm for 4 mm lesions.

Stage IV (AJCC) Surgery if possible, even though there is little prospect of cure. Metastasectomy is not normally recommended, apart from symptomatic metastases of the GI tract, because of the short median survival.

Radiotherapy Cutaneous melanoma is relatively resistant.
- Superficial lesions occasionally treated with this modality.
- Postoperative irradiation of affected lymph node sites increases the risk of lymphoedema without increasing the cure rate.

Chemotherapy Melanoma is one of the more chemoresistant tumours. Soft tissue and skin metastases respond better than do lung or other visceral/CNS secondaries. Median duration of response is around 6 months. High-dose chemotherapy has not been shown to increase the response duration.

- Dacarbazine (DTIC) — one of the most active agents, with a single agent activity of 15–25%.
- Nitrosoureas and platinums also have single-agent activity of around 20%, with little evidence of synergistic activity with combination therapy.

Immunotherapy The evidence that melanocytes have receptors for several GFs raised hopes that the newer immunological and biological therapies would achieve an increase in response rate. Interferons and interleukins were initially thought to achieve response rates of 20%, and combination therapies with chemo-immunotherapies continue but without clear evidence of improved activity.

Recurrent disease

Local relapse • Within 5 cm of the scar of the initial lesion — approximately 3% within the first 5 years. • Resection with a generous excision margin, where possible.

Multiple local or in-transit lesions • Laser therapy • Isolated limb perfusion using melphalan.

Relapse in a regional lymph node site • Radical lymph-node dissection.

Metastatic disease

Stage IV There may be a time lag of over 20 years between resection of the primary and development of metastases. In these cases, biopsy of the metastatic lesion is mandatory. CNS secondaries are found in 20% of patients.

Prognosis (→ Table 4.31)

TABLE 4.31 Survival related to number of metastatic sites		
Number of metastatic sites	**Median survival (months)**	**1-year survival**
Single	7	36%
2 sites	4	13%
≥ 3 sites	2	0%

AJCC stage I–II disease
- Site of disease is significant with survival in upper limb > lower limb > trunk or head and neck.
- Scalp lesions are the worst in head and neck melanoma.
- Women survive longer than men (? related to higher frequency of primaries on the limbs).
- Tumour thickness (vertical height) is the single most important prognostic indicator, survival being inversely related to the level of invasion (10-year mortality rate 30% for 2 mm vs 70% for 6 mm).
- Ulceration indicates an aggressive, bad-prognosis lesion.
- Lentigo maligna melanomas carry a better prognosis.

AJCC stage III disease
The number of metastatic nodes is the clearest predictor for survival. 5-year survival with one node: 60%; with 2–4 nodes, 25%; with > 5 nodes, 10%.

AJCC Stage IV disease (→ Table 4.32)

TABLE 4.32 AJCC stage IV disease

Site of first relapse	% patients	Median survival
Skin, distant nodes, subcutaneous tissue	60	7 months
Lung	35	11 months
Brain, bones, liver	5	2–6 months

SQUAMOUS CELL CARCINOMA

SCC of the skin is often well differentiated and can be recognized by the production of keratin, which results in a warty, scaly lesion.

Risk factors
Solar keratosis • Typically on hands and face exposed to sunlight • 65–75 year age group, or 30 years of age for fair-skinned populations of tropical climates.

Leukoplakia • Mucous membrane equivalent of solar keratosis, caused by chronic irritation from smoking, poor hygiene, syphilis • A small proportion progresses to SCC • Affecting lips, oral cavity, vulva.

Bowen's disease Slowly progressive intra-epidermal carcinoma which often resembles a patch of psoriasis or eczema. It tends to run an indolent course.

Making the diagnosis

- Regular surveillance of predisposing lesions.
- Complete excision of leukoplakia if possible.
- Excision of patches of Bowen's disease to prevent invasive carcinoma from developing.
- Biopsy is essential to differentiate from solar keratosis and leukoplakia and from basal cell carcinoma and keratoacanthoma. Differentiation of keratoacanthoma from SCC is difficult and excision biopsy or curettage is the correct treatment.
- Palpation of the regional lymph nodes for involvement if the diagnosis has been made late or the lesion is poorly differentiated.
- FNAC of suspicious nodes for assessment.

Differential diagnosis

Basal cell carcinoma See below.

Keratoacanthoma Benign condition arising on the face and hands characterized by rapid proliferation of squamous epidermal cells. These tumours grow very rapidly to attain a size of 2 cm within 6 weeks, often with a keratin plug filling the centre of the dome-shaped nodule. The lesion then gradually involutes to leave a depressed scar.

Treatment

If the diagnosis has been obtained by excision biopsy with a clear margin then no further treatment may be necessary, particularly for well-differentiated tumours in the elderly.

As a general rule: • surgical block dissection for mobile nodes • regional radiotherapy for fixed nodes.

BASAL CELL CARCINOMA

BCC is mostly seen in the skin of the face and neck. Tumours are often slow growing, but can penetrate deeper tissues such as cartilage and bone if left untreated. Metastases are rare, but death can occur from sepsis following penetration of the skull or orbit.

Risk factors

- Sunlight exposure.
- Age > 50 years.

Making the diagnosis

- Early lesion is often soft, smooth and translucent.
- Later lesion develops a central ulcerated depression with a surrounding rolled edge.

Treatment
Excision biopsy to obtain clear deep and lateral margins.

- Larger lesions:
  — preliminary small biopsy
  — post biopsy, fractionated course of radiotherapy.
- Recurrent and larger neglected lesions may require extensive operation to obtain clear margins:
  — resection of involved bone and cartilage
  — frozen section biopsy confirmation of clearance
  — repair of defect with myocutaneous flaps.

CARCINOMA OF THE LUNG

Lung cancer is the commonest cause of cancer death in the UK with only a minimal improvement in 5-year survival in the past 15 years. It is increasing in incidence among women. Prognosis and treatment protocols vary according to whether the histology is a 'small cell lung cancer' (25%) or a 'non-small cell lung cancer' (75%).

Risk factors
Caused by smoking in 90% of cases.

Staging (→ Table 4.33)

TABLE 4.33 Carcinoma of the lung: staging

T1	≤ 3 cm
T2	> 3 cm, involving hilar region/visceral pleura/with partial atelectasis
T3	Invades adjacent structures, e.g. chest wall, diaphragm, pericardium, mediastinal pleura/with total atelectasis
a	With limited node involvement
b	With extensive node involvement
T4	Invades mediastinum, heart, great vessels, trachea, oesophagus, carina; malignant pleural effusion
N1	Ipsilateral peribronchial/hilar lymph nodes
N2	Ipsilateral mediastinal/subcarinal lymph nodes
N3	Contralateral regional lymph nodes

Making the diagnosis
Signs and symptoms • Chronic cough • Dyspnoea • Recurrent pneumonia • Haemoptysis • Pain • Abnormality on a routine CXR • Unexplained hyponatraemia • Hoarse voice.

Investigations • CXR • Sputum cytology • Bronchoscopy with biopsy is the definitive investigation • CT scan to assess resectability of NSCLC.

Histology
• NSCLC squamous cell (epidermoid), adenocarcinoma, large cell: 75%.
• SCLC: 25%.

Treatment
Dependent on cell type, stage and patient's performance status.

Small cell lung cancer (SCLC)

This is generally believed to be a systemic disease by the time of diagnosis, and is very rarely resectable. Cure rates for resection of small tumours are reported, but only 5% are early tumours and generally systemic treatment with chemotherapy is the optimum treatment. Adjuvant chemotherapy should be given if a lung tumour resected as a diagnostic and therapeutic procedure is found to be small cell cancer with nodal involvement.

Without therapy, the survival is around 3 months. Treatment is with combination chemotherapy (e.g. adriamycin, cyclophosphamide and etoposide—'ACE') which achieves response rates of 80% and complete responses in around 60% of patients. Those patients with limited disease who achieve complete response should have consolidative irradiation to the site of the primary tumour, since this significantly increases the relapse-free period.

Patients of poor performance status may respond better to combination chemotherapy than single agent treatment (e.g. oral etoposide) but four rather than six cycles only should be prescribed. If a patient is symptomatic from the primary tumour but unfit for chemotherapy, local radiotherapy is an effective treatment with the understanding that it will have no effect on the metastatic sites of disease.

Approximately 30% of patients with SCLC develop brain metastases, and prophylactic cranial irradiation may be of benefit for those who are fit and who achieve CR.

The majority of patients relapse within 1 year and no benefit from maintenance chemotherapy or alpha interferon has been demonstrated.

The 2-year survival for good prognosis patients is around 20% and < 5% for those with adverse prognostic factors.

Bad prognostic factors in SCLC

- Extensive disease (present outwith one hemithorax)
- WHO performance status > 2
- Liver and bone marrow metastases
- Elevated LDH
- Raised alkaline phosphatase
- Male sex

Non-small cell lung cancer (NSCLC)

Only 20% of patients with this tumour present with disease at a resectable stage (T1, T2 or occasionally T3a). Surgery offers the best prospect of cure, but even in those with stage I disease the 5-year survival is around 60%. Patients may die of local or distant relapse, or may succumb to other smoking-related disorders (cardiovascular disease, second tumours). Most thoracic surgeons are reluctant to resect disease at stage T3a, and these tumours are conventionally treated with local and mediastinal irradiation.

Radical radiotherapy can produce durable remissions in a select group of patients with early stage disease.

The role of preoperative chemotherapy in operable (stage T1 and T2) or borderline operable (stage T3a) NSCLC is currently being investigated in large randomized trials.

The median survival for patients with more advanced tumours is in the order of 8 months. Conventionally, local and regional irradiation has been the treatment of choice.

Increasing interest is now being shown in combination chemotherapy either in addition to or instead of radiotherapy for more advanced disease in NSCLC. Combinations such as mitomycin-C, ifosfamide and cisplatin (MIC) or mitomycin-C, vinblastine and cisplatin (MVP) achieve objective response rates of around 50% in locally advanced disease, and symptomatic responses in 70% of patients, equivalent to that seen with radiotherapy.

Assessment of the patients' quality of life on treatment with an experimental chemotherapy (whether single agent or combination) or with radiotherapy is an important part of such studies. Several of the newer chemotherapies (e.g. taxol, gemcitabine) demonstrate a response rate of around 30% in NSCLC and their use in combination will be a central part of future studies in this disease.

MESOTHELIOMA

This malignant tumour of the pleura is linked to asbestos exposure, and there is usually extensive pleural involvement by the time of diagnosis. It tends to be unresponsive to chemotherapy and has a poor prognosis.

CENTRAL NERVOUS SYSTEM TUMOURS

Tumours of the central nervous system comprise 2–7% of all primary tumours, and 20% of childhood cancers. The peak age incidence occurs between 5 and 10 years and between 50 and 60 years. Primary intracranial tumours spread by local infiltration. Lymphatic spread is virtually unheard of and vascular metastases are exceedingly rare. The higher-grade tumours can, however, 'seed' into the subarachnoid and ventricular spaces. The most common malignant brain tumour is a secondary deposit.

Primary tumours	
Astrocytoma	60%
Ependymoma	6%
Oligodendroglioma	6%
Meningioma	10%
Pineal	5%

Risk factors
- Increased incidence associated with
  — tuberous sclerosis
  — von Recklinghausen's disease
  — von Hippel–Lindau disease.
- Environmental factors (aromatic hydrocarbons).
- Viruses.
- Cranial irradiation.

Making the diagnosis
Signs and symptoms Commonest symptoms: • headache • convulsion • altered mental function • focal neurological deficit.
Raised ICP: • early morning headache • vomiting • papilloedema • hypertension • bradycardia • decreased conscious level.

Investigations • Imaging—CT or MR scanning • Biopsy, excision, CSF examination for histological confirmation • Biochemical and endocrine profile • Where cerebral metastases are suspected, appropriate investigations for primary tumour, e.g. CXR.

ASTROCYTOMA

The treatment and prognosis of astrocytomas depend primarily on their surgical resectability, and also on their histological grade (high grade or low grade).

Making the diagnosis
- Initial assessment should involve a neurosurgical opinion.
- Histological confirmation by CSF cytology or biopsy, including stereotactic biopsy where appropriate.

Histology
- High grade.
- Low grade.

Treatment
Dexamethasone reduces cerebral oedema and should be considered for all patients with raised ICP or focal neurological signs.

Surgery Stereotactic biopsy now permits tissue diagnosis from regions of the brain previously considered inaccessible (e.g. brain stem). For resectable tumours, debulking should be as complete as possible, providing a dead space to accommodate recurrence. Repeat surgical excision should be considered for low-grade tumours, particularly with prolonged disease-free interval. It is rarely beneficial for high-grade tumours.

Radiotherapy
Low-grade Should be considered for unresectable tumours and where surgical excision was not complete, to reduce subsequent recurrence rates.

High-grade Should be restricted to patients with limited neurological deficit and good performance status.

Chemotherapy CCNU, a lipophylic agent capable of crossing the blood–brain barrier, is the basis of chemotherapy for high-grade tumours. Response rates of 30–40% have been reported, but in most cases responses are short-lived.

Prognosis
5-year survival for low grade is 50% and for high grade 5%.
Factors influencing prognosis include:

- histological grade
- degree of neurological deficit
- completeness of surgery
- age < 40
- site of tumour (e.g. brain stem carries a poor prognosis).

MENINGIOMA

Meningioma represents 15–20% of primary intracranial tumours. The majority of these very slow-growing tumours are benign, and the average interval to recurrence following surgical excision is 4 years. The most common sites are the parasagittal falx region, the cerebral convexities and the sphenoid ridge. Patients may present with epilepsy, headache or focal neurological signs.

Treatment

Surgery Excision is the mainstay of treatment.

Radiotherapy Limited to those patients in whom surgical excision was incomplete, or in cases of repeated recurrence.

Prognosis

For most patients, very good.

MEDULLOBLASTOMA

These tumours arise from primitive neuroepithelial cells in the roof of the fourth ventricle. They most commonly present in childhood and adolescence and account for 4–8% of all primary brain tumours and 25% of intracranial tumours in childhood.

Signs and symptoms Patients present with symptoms including dizziness, nystagmus, headache, vomiting, truncal ataxia, raised ICP or focal neurology.

Treatment

Surgery Excision should be attempted unless the site and size of the tumour make this hazardous.

Radiotherapy Encompasses the primary tumour and spinal cord.

Chemotherapy May improve survival, but this has not yet been confirmed.

Prognosis

40–60% of patients alive and well at 5 years. Poor prognostic features include:

- gross neurological symptoms and signs
- incomplete surgical excision
- age < 15 years
- presentation with spinal metastases.

OLIGODENDROGLIOMA

Oligodendroglioma usually appears in the fifth decade of life. These tumours are confined to supratentorial regions of the brain and 40% show calcification. Spinal seedlings are rare. Other characteristics include:

- 2/3 of tumours occur in the frontal lobe
- 2/3 of patients have a preceding history of at least 5 years
- 2/3 of patients present with epilepsy
- 2/3 of patients are amenable to good subtotal resection
- 2/3 of patients have raised ICP
- 2/3 of patients survive 5 years.

Treatment

Surgery Complete excision should be attempted.

Radiotherapy Indicated in cases where surgical excision is incomplete.

Chemotherapy Occasionally used in high-grade disease on recurrence.

Prognosis
60–80% 5-year survival.

EPENDYMOMA

These tumours are derived from ependymal cells lining the ventricles and central canal of the spinal cord. They usually occur in adolescents and young adults and comprise 60% of primary spinal cord gliomas. High-grade and infratentorial tumours have a propensity for seeding via CSF.

Histology
- High grade.
- Low grade.

Treatment
Surgery May involve a posterior fossa craniectomy or spinal cord decompression. Excision should be as complete as possible.

Radiotherapy
Low grade Wide field treatment to the tumour bed.

High grade and infratentorial Whole CNS radiotherapy

Chemotherapy The place of CCNU chemotherapy in high-grade disease on recurrence remains unclear.

Prognosis
- *50–60% 5-year survival*—late relapse very unusual.
- Low grade: median survival 10 years.
- High grade: median survival 2–3 years.

BONE TUMOURS

OSTEOGENIC SARCOMA

Osteogenic sarcoma is the commonest of the primary malignant bone
tumours and occurs more frequently in males. It primarily arises in the
metaphysis of long tubular bones (distal femur, proximal tibia, proximal
fibula, proximal humerus).

Risk factors
- Age — occurs predominantly between 10 and 20 years of age.
- Rarely — can arise as a complication of Paget's disease of bone in later life.

Staging (→ Table 4.34)

TABLE 4.34 Osteogenic sarcoma: staging

T1	Within cortex
T2	Invades beyond cortex
N1	Regional lymph node involvement

Making the diagnosis
Signs and symptoms • A bony swelling around the knee or shoulder in an
adolescent should be assumed to be an osteosarcoma until proven otherwise
• Pain • Limp • Effusion • Typical radiological appearances of Codman's
triangle (caused by the periosteum laying down new bone as it is peeled off
the bone cortex by the expanding tumour) and 'sun ray' spicules (caused by
new bone formation within the soft tissues invaded by the expanding tumour).

Investigations • X-ray of the affected limb • CXR • Open biopsy —
needle biopsies, e.g. TruCut, are not sufficiently reliable to establish the
diagnosis confidently and open biopsies are usually preferred. The incision
must be chosen so that the scar can be excised in continuity with the tumour
if the diagnosis is confirmed. Best performed by the specialist team who will
perform the definitive surgery. • CT scan of lungs — commonest site of
metastatic disease • Isotope bone scan • CT or MR scan of the tumour for
extent of local invasion.

Differential diagnosis
Includes: • osteomyelitis • benign aneurysmal bone cyst • giant cell
tumour • Ewing's sarcoma • post-traumatic myositis ossificans.

Treatment

Chemotherapy First treatment modality for most patients, achieving significant regression of the primary tumour in over 80%. Effective drugs include: • adriamycin • cisplatin • methotrexate • vincristine • ifosfamide.

Surgery On completion of chemotherapy, the tumour is reassessed for operability.

- Limb-conserving resection of the involved bone with implantation of long-stemmed movable endoprosthesis in the hip, knee or shoulder can be performed in the majority of patients.
- Amputation above the level of the affected bone for locally non-resectable cases, provided that no distant metastases have been demonstrated on repeated staging investigations.
- 5%–10% of patients may develop local recurrence following initially successful limb-preserving primary treatment.

Metastatic disease

- Chemotherapy may achieve useful responses and should be recommended, particularly if the metastatic disease is symptomatic.
- Long-term survival is only possible if lung metastases are resectable, and the advice of a thoracic surgeon should be sought.
- Best results are seen with solitary or a small number of metastases confined to one lung.

Prognosis

Overall survival at 5 years is 40%. This compares to about 15% in the days prior to the introduction of pre-operative chemotherapy.

SOFT TISSUE SARCOMAS

Soft tissue sarcomas account for about 1% of adult malignancies, and arise from connective tissue anywhere in the body. Limbs and limb girdles are common sites.

Risk factors
Neurofibromatosis Carries an approximate 10% lifetime risk of sarcoma (usually MPNST).

Radiation-induced sarcomas May occur several years after radiotherapy for another condition, e.g. breast cancer, and are particularly difficult to treat.

Making the diagnosis
* CT/MR scan (unless the lump is very superficial).
* TruCut needle biopsy
  — to establish tumour grade: tumour behaviour tends to correlate more with grade than with histological subtype
  — to confirm tumour type, i.e. that it is a soft tissue sarcoma; that it is not a lymphoma or carcinoma.
* CT scan of the lungs to exclude metastases.

> ⚠️ Do not proceed directly to surgical removal: a simple 'shell-out'
> excision is insufficient despite apparent encapsulation. The tumour
> may be extensive; there is the risk of an inappropriately sited scar; and a useful
> pre-operative CT/MR scan of the lesion will be impossible.

Differential diagnosis
Distinguish soft tissue sarcoma from: • embryonal sarcoma or Ewing's sarcoma (they are chemosensitive) • bone tumours (treatment protocols are different) • desmoid tumour (see pp. 144–145) • Kaposi's sarcoma (see p. 164).

Common histological subtypes of adult soft-tissue sarcoma
Malignant fibrous histiocytoma (MFH)
Liposarcoma
Malignant peripheral nerve sheath tumour (MPNST)
Synovial sarcoma
Sarcoma NOS (not otherwise specified)
Epithelioid sarcoma
Fibrosarcoma
Chondrosarcoma
Leiomyosarcoma

Treatment

Primary tumour
Treatment is usually a combination of optimal surgery with adjuvant radiotherapy.

- Compartmentectomy
    — the important principle is to remove 1 uninvolved tissue plane in all directions around tumour
    — for limb sarcomas, involved muscles removed from origin to insertion
    — reconstruction of defect using a pedicled or free flap with microvascular anastomosis may be required in 10–20% of cases.
- Major amputation
    — reserved only for those tumours (often recurrent) where surgical removal cannot be achieved by any other means.
- Radical postoperative radiotherapy to tumour bed and associated compartment once wounds are healed.
- Preoperative radiotherapy, preferred in some centres, is particularly useful to shrink rapidly growing bulky tumours before resection.
- Follow-up includes regular CXR as distant metastases occur in the lungs.

As yet there is no good data to support the routine use of adjuvant and neoadjuvant chemotherapy.

Metastatic disease
Surgery Metastasectomy for a solitary or small number of resectable metastases in an otherwise fit patient.

Chemotherapy For multiple metastases, can give a useful response but is best reserved for symptomatic disease. Active agents are adriamycin, epirubicin and ifosfamide.

Prognosis
5-year survival after optimal therapy of primary sarcomas: low grade 70%, high grade 40%.

RETROPERITONEAL SARCOMA

Retroperitoneal sarcomas represent a particularly difficult clinical problem. The only realistic hope of cure for these tumours lies in successful surgical clearance. Multiple organ involvement reduces the likelihood that the tumour will be resectable.

Making the diagnosis
Signs and symptoms • Usually presents as abdominal mass, often of large volume • Characteristic appearances on CT scan.

Investigations • Examination of lymph node areas and testes • CT scan: image sarcoma, assess involvement of ureters and other organs • Percutaneous biopsy under CT or ultrasound guidance where diagnosis is unclear.

Differential diagnosis
Includes:

- retroperitoneal lymphoma
- teratoma
- carcinoma (e.g. pancreas or kidney).

Treatment
Surgery • Laparotomy and 'trial dissection' to see if macroscopic tumour clearance can be achieved • Complete resection of primary tumour with resection of involved organs in continuity if necessary.

Radiotherapy Adjuvant to surgery where technically feasible, it is rarely possible because of the large volume of tumours and the proximity of spinal cord, kidneys and bowel.

Chemotherapy Palliative treatment of symptomatic lung metastasis only.

Prognosis
- Apparently complete macroscopic resection: 50% 5-year survival.
- Incompletely resected low-grade tumours of indolent natural history: 20% 5-year survival.
- Incompletely resected high-grade tumours: 0% 5-year survival.
- > 80% risk of local recurrence, particularly for high-grade tumours.

> ⚠ In young adults with a retroperitoneal sarcoma, consideration should be given to a trial of chemotherapy before surgery, since some will have an embryonal type of sarcoma which is chemosensitive. If a CT response is seen after 2 courses of chemotherapy in e.g. Ewing's sarcoma (see pp. 148–149), the chemotherapy can be continued until maximal response and then residual disease can be resected.

DESMOID TUMOURS

Desmoid tumours (otherwise known as fibromatosis) are not true sarcomas since they do not metastasize, but their behaviour in local tissues is very similar and the principles of management are the same. They often occur in young adults associated with familial adenomatous polyposis (Gardner's syndrome).

They occasionally cause death through aggressive local invasion of vital structures. For desmoids that are non-resectable or recurrent after previous surgery and radiotherapy, useful responses have been reported with tamoxifen, toremifene and prolonged low-dose chemotherapy.

DERMATOFIBROSARCOMA PROTUBERANS (DFP)

DFP is a cutaneous sarcoma with a remarkable propensity for local recurrence unless wide clearance (e.g. 5 cm of skin) is taken. Metastases have not been observed.

SOLID PAEDIATRIC TUMOURS

After trauma, cancer is the commonest cause of death in children under the age of 15 years, accounting for 700 deaths every year in Britain. The most common paediatric cancers are listed below:

- 25% leukaemia (80% ALL) — see pages 158–163.
- 20% brain — see pages 136–139.
- 10% lymphoma — see pages 150–155.
- 8% neuroblastoma
- 8% sarcoma
- 7% nephroblastoma.

Germ cell and epithelial tumours form the majority of the remainder.

There is a much improved cure rate in paediatric tumours (50%) compared with adult cancers. This is directly attributable to the higher proportion of ALL and the relatively recent increase in cure of these malignancies. It is very important that paediatric cancers are treated in or closely supervised by a specialist paediatric cancer unit, both to ensure optimum treatment (often in study protocols) and to enable parents to obtain maximum support during the child's treatment and follow-up period.

The difference between treating a paediatric as opposed to an adult cancer lies not only in the higher likelihood of cure but also in the long term side-effects of cancer treatment. Exposure of immature bones to radiotherapy can result in asymmetrical growth with attendant cosmetic and structural problems. Chemotherapy may induce sterility in both male and female children.

The incidence of second tumours is also very relevant in this patient population, and the recent publications on the potential of etoposide to cause leukaemia have again emphasised the importance of monitoring the long-term effects of potentially curative treatment regimens. Patients who have received MOPP chemotherapy to treat Hodgkin's disease have a 4% incidence of AML within the 10 years after treatment.

NEUROBLASTOMA

Neuroblastoma is a tumour which can arise anywhere along the sympathetic nervous system. It is the most common solid tumour of childhood outside of the central nervous system. 50% of these tumours occur by the age of 2 years with a slight preponderance of females. Distant bone metastases are present in 45% of children. Spontaneous remission is most common in the youngest children and cure is directly proportional to the age of the child at diagnosis. The survival rate is around 90% at 2 years in children with early stage disease (no tumour across the midline and no distant metastatic disease) but falls to 30% with more advanced stages.

Making the diagnosis
Signs and symptoms A tender mass is the most common presenting symptom but 25% of tumours produce no symptoms. The stage of disease is established with a combination of IVU (displacement of entire kidney and collecting system), ultrasound, bone scan and CT scan. There may be calcification within the mass.

Treatment
Treatment is with surgical excision in as many cases as possible, even if the tumour seems to be advanced. Post-operative radiotherapy and chemotherapy will be indicated if complete removal is not possible or if the neuroblastoma is advanced at diagnosis. Vincristine, cisplatin, doxorubicin and cyclophosphamide/ifosfamide are effective drugs in this tumour type.

Radiotherapy is especially useful in palliation of painful bone metastases.

WILM'S TUMOUR (NEPHROBLASTOMA)

Up to 80% of these congenital, embryonal renal cell neoplasms occur before the age of 5 years. Bilateral disease is present in 5–10% of cases.

Making the diagnosis
Symptoms and signs A 'silent' abdominal mass is the commonest presentation. Haematuria or hypertension are present in 25% of patients. Metastases are most often found in the lungs. Bone marrow involvement is rare.

Investigation IVU, ultrasound, CT scan and CXR are central investigations in establishing the stage of the tumour when histological diagnosis has been established.

Treatment
Treatment is primarily surgical since the tumour is often encapsulated. Biopsy of the contralateral kidney is recommended. Unilateral and contralateral partial nephrectomy may be necessary. Post-operative chemotherapy with drug combinations including vincristine, doxorubicin, cyclophosphamide and dactinomycin is usually required.

Prognosis
Even children with pulmonary metastases may be cured, with a reported success rate of 50% following a combination of surgery, radiotherapy and chemotherapy.

SOFT TISSUE SARCOMAS

Rhabdomyosarcoma is the commonest soft tissue sarcoma in childhood. The peak incidence is between 2 and 5 years of age with 70% of children presenting before the age of 10 years. The male to female ratio is 1.4:1.

Making the diagnosis
The commonest site of presentation is head and neck (38%), genitourinary area (21%) or extremity (18%). The tumour has a predisposition for the orbit, causing bruising (may be mistaken for non-accidental injury), proptosis or ocular paralysis.

Treatment
Treatment is primarily by surgical excision aiming for complete remission (stage I disease), removal of all macroscopic disease (stage II) or debulking of the local disease only (stage III). Disant metastases confer stage IV status. In all cases radiotherapy and chemotherapy increase the cure rate from the 15% achieved following surgery alone.

Prognosis
Patients with stage III disease who achieve complete remission have a 5-year survival rate of 60% compared with 30% for stage IV disease.

EWING'S SARCOMA

First described in 1920, the radiosensitivity of Ewing's sarcoma differentiates it from other sarcomas.

Treatment
The problem of treatment is typical of many tumours in that local relapse is followed by dissemination to other sites; only 10% recur locally alone. Combined chemotherapy, surgery and radiotherapy is the treatment of choice, with chemotherapy always given first to facilitate resection and possibly to 'mop up' micrometastases. Vincristine, adriamycin, cyclophosphamide, ifosfamide and actinomycin are active agents.

There is no evidence of a dose/response curve after giving more than 50 Gy radiotherapy, but 40–60 Gy are usually given postoperatively where there is incomplete resection or microscopic residual disease.

Prognosis (→ Table 4.35)

TABLE 4.35 Ewing's sarcoma: prognosis	
Depends on	Stage of disease: worse with metastases at diagnosis.
	Axial long bone involvement worse than distal long bone, worse than proximal long bone.
	Old age (worse)
	Male sex (worse)
Survival	For all patients with local disease: around 50% at 5 years

HAEMATOLOGICAL MALIGNANCIES

HODGKIN'S DISEASE

Hodgkin's disease has a bimodal age distribution with peak incidence between 18 and 35 years and 55 and 70 years. There is a slight female preponderance. The uniform pattern of lymph node involvement is reflected in the staging system and the approach to treatment.

Risk factors
• Infections agents implicated, e.g. EBV.

Staging (→ Table 4.36)

TABLE 4.36 Hodgkin's disease: staging	
Ann Arbor system	
Stage I	Involvement of I lymph node area or a single extralymphatic organ or site (I_E)
Stage II	> I lymph node area involved on the same side of the diaphragm or localized involvement of extralymphatic organ and one or more lymph node regions on the same side of the diaphragm (II_E)
Stage III	Nodal disease on both sides of the diaphragm or with extra lymphatic site (III_E) or spleen (III_S)
Stage IV	Involvement of extranodal sites e.g. bone marrow (IV_M), liver (IV_H), lung (IV_L)
B symptoms	
• Night sweats	
• Fever > 38°C for 3 consecutive days	
• Unexplained weight loss of > 10% body weight	

Making the diagnosis
Signs and symptoms • Painless soft mobile lymph node, usually in the neck • Fatigue • Pruritus • Alcohol-induced nodal pain (occasionally) • History of repeated infective episodes • Mediastinal adenopathy on CXR • Persistent cough • Splenomegaly.

Investigations • Palpation of all lymph node areas + abdomen for hepatosplenomegaly • Lymph node biopsy • FBC and ESR • Biochemical profile including liver enzymes, serum lactate dehydrogenase (LDH) and B_2 microglobulin • CXR • CT scan thorax, abdomen, pelvis • Bone marrow aspirate and trephine • Fertility counselling and sperm banking if appropriate.

Histology
Characterized by the presence of multinucleated giant cells —
Reed–Sternberg cells.

Major histological categories
- Nodular sclerosing 70%.
- Lymphocyte predominant 15%.
- Lymphocyte depleted 5%.
- Mixed cell 10%.

Treatment

Stage I – II without B symptoms
Involved field radiotherapy for 4–6 weeks.

Stage IB and IIB – IVB
Combination chemotherapy, occasionally followed by local radiation to sites
of initial bulk disease.

Chemotherapy
1. MOPP—mustine, vincristine, procarbazine, prednisolone, or
2. ABVD—adriamycin, bleomycin, vinblastine, DTIC, or
3. CHIVPP—chlorambucil, vinblastine, procarbazine, prednisolone, or
4. VEEP—vincristine, epirubicin, etoposide, prednisolone (preserved gonadal
   function).

High-dose chemotherapy usually with peripheral blood stem cell rescue in
high-risk ± relapse patients.

Prognosis
Factors associated with poorer prognosis are: • increasing stage of disease
• B symptoms • age > 40 years • bulk disease (particularly mediastinal
bulk adenopathy) • lymphocyte-depleted histological subtype—high LDH,
ESR ± B_2 microglobulin. Most relapses occur in the first 1–2 years following
completion of therapy.

Stage I and IIA disease
- Radiotherapy-treated—relapse rate approximately 25%.
- Subsequent combination chemotherapy—virtually 100% cure.

Stage III and IV disease ± B symptoms
- Overall 60% disease-free at 5 years.
- Variations depend on the number of adverse prognostic factors.

Treatment at relapse
- If < 12 months since first treatment, non-cross-resistant chemotherapy ± radiotherapy, then high-dose chemotherapy with bone marrow rescue.
- If > 12 months since first treatment, non-cross-resistant chemotherapy ± radiotherapy.

NON-HODGKIN'S LYMPHOMA

For the purpose of clinical course and treatment strategy, non-Hodgkin's lymphoma (NHL) may be subdivided into:

1. high- and intermediate-grade NHL
2. low-grade NHL.

HIGH- AND INTERMEDIATE-GRADE NHL

This disease spans from childhood to old age with a median age at presentation of 50–60 years. It affects approximately 2500 people each year in the UK, with an equal gender distribution. It is characterized by rapid onset, with 60–70% of patients presenting with disseminated disease (stages III and IV). In most cases the disease originates in a lymph node area and spreads within the lymphoreticular system. About 25–30% of patients show extranodal spread typically to bone marrow, liver and lung. Primary extranodal NHL occurs in 15–20% of cases, usually involving the GI tract, less commonly bone, lung, skin and brain.

Risk factors
Impaired immune surveillance, e.g. post renal/cardiac transplantation, treatment for malignancy (Hodgkin's disease) AIDS. (See AIDS-related cancer, pp. 164–165).

Staging
As for Hodgkin's disease.

Making the diagnosis
Signs and symptoms ● Short history of palpable lymph node enlargement, usually associated with a degree of lethargy ● B symptoms may be present ● Respiratory symptoms if significant mediastinal adenopathy or lung parenchymal involvement ● Abdominal symptoms and low back pain — may herald intra-abdominal adenopathy ● Systemic consequences of advanced disease: impaired marrow function, renal failure ● Pallor and weight loss — more advanced disease.

Investigations • Examination of all lymph node areas • Assessment for hepatosplenomegaly • Lymph node biopsy • FBC and ESR • Biochemistry profile including liver enzymes, serum lactate dehydrogenase (LDH) and B_2 microglobulin (B_2M) • CXR • CT scan thorax, abdomen and pelvis • Bone marrow aspirate and trephine biopsy • Lumbar puncture if immunoblastic, lymphoblastic, marrow involvement or primarily testicular.

Histology

Classifications most commonly adopted in Europe are the Working Formulation and the Kiel classification:

- characterized by a loss of follicular lymph node architecture
- individual subtypes defined by the cytological appearance of the predominant malignant cell type (refer to a specialized text for details).

Treatment

Combination chemotherapy is the treatment of choice for all patients irrespective of tumour stage. Locoregional radiotherapy alone is given:

- for small-volume stage IA
- particularly when the patient is frail and likely to experience difficulty with chemotherapy.

Radiotherapy May be used to treat sites of prior bulk disease on completion of the course of chemotherapy.

Chemotherapy Standard CHOP regimen (cyclophosphamide, doxorubicin, vincristine and prednisolone) administered on a 3-weekly cycle for 4–6 months. Weekly chemotherapy regimens are not proven to be superior to conventional CHOP therapy.

For patients with a poor prognosis:

- high-dose cytotoxic therapy with bone marrow support
  — conventional bone marrow transplantation techniques
  — bone marrow reconstitution using peripheral blood stem cells harvested following stimulation with haemopoietic growth factors, e.g. granulocyte colony-stimulating factor (GCSF).

Recurrent disease

Most relapses occur in the first 1–2 years following completion of therapy.

Prognosis

Factors associated with poorer prognosis:

- increasing stage of disease
- poor performance status at presentation
- tumour burden, as estimated by the presence of large nodal masses, *or* biochemical parameters, e.g. serum LDH.

Disease free at 5 years:

- Stage I–II: 70%
- Stage III–IV: 40%.

LOW-GRADE NHL
There are approximately 1000 new cases in the UK each year. It is rare below the age of 40 and has an equal gender distribution. The disease may be insidious in onset and is usually widespread at diagnosis. It runs an indolent yet persistent course.

Risk factors
- Associated with Bcl 2 gene expression.
- Many tumours carry a 14:8 translocation.

Staging
As for Hodgkin's disease.

Making the diagnosis
Signs and symptoms • Persistent disseminated lymph node enlargement • History of frequent infective episodes due to disease-associated immune impairment • Symptoms caused by anaemia or thrombocytopenia due to heavy bone marrow infiltration or hypersplenism • Abdominal discomfort and distension due to significant splenomegaly and, to a lesser extent, hepatomegaly • Sweats, weight loss and lethargy—common systemic symptoms.

Investigations • Lymph node biopsy • FBC and ESR • Biochemistry profile including liver enzymes and serum lactate dehydrogenase (LDH) • CXR • CT scan • Bone marrow aspirate and trephine biopsy.

Histology
Characterized by the preservation of the follicular lymph node architecture. Exception is diffuse lymphocytic lymphoma which is also included in this category.

Treatment
Stage IA Complete surgical excision followed by locoregional radiotherapy.

Disseminated disease
- Asymptomatic (without a large tumour burden): observation with no therapy (eventual outcome is independent of how early therapy is initiated).
- More advanced symptomatic disease: chemotherapy ± radiation.

Chemotherapy • Oral alkylating agents: chlorambucil administered intermittently on a monthly cycle for 6–12 months • IV chemotherapy if response to chlorambucil is unsatisfactory: combination therapy, e.g. CVP (cyclophosphamide, vincristine and prednisolone), CHOP or single-agent therapy, e.g. fludarabine • High-dose therapy with bone marrow rescue for highly resistant disease is being evaluated in clinical trials.

Radiotherapy • Total nodal irradiation • Modified large field techniques using relatively low doses of radiation—less commonly employed in recent years • Local radiotherapy for enlarged nodes which have responded poorly to chemotherapy, and to areas of initial bulky disease as consolidation after chemotherapy to reduce the risk of local recurrent disease

Interferon-α 50% response rate when administered alone. A number of clinical studies have suggested that its major role may lie in delaying relapse if administered after completion of chemotherapy.

Prognosis
Stage IA Very uncommon; treatment offers the potential for cure.

Disseminated Incurable disease with chronic relapsing pattern and median survival of 7–10 years.

Sequelae
Chemotherapy Administration becomes progressively more difficult due to poor bone marrow reserve as a consequence of marrow infiltration and the effects of long-term administration of bone marrow-damaging drugs.

Interferon-α Side-effects include fatigue, fever and flu-like symptoms.

MYELOMA

Myeloma accounts for 1% of all neoplasms. It is more common in older people (median age 69 in men, 71 in women) but rare in people < 40 years old (2% of cases). The disease spectrum ranges from monoclonal gammopathy to plasma cell leukaemia. Myeloma is not a curable disease.

Risk factors
• Associated with exposure to radiation.

Staging (→ Table 4.37)

TABLE 4.37 Myeloma: staging	
Major criteria*	
I	Plasmacytoma on tissue biopsy
II	Bone marrow plasmacytosis with > 30% plasma cells
III	Monoclonal globulin spike on serum electrophoresis
	> 3.5 g/dl for IgG, > 30 g/dl for IgA
	≥ 1.0 g/24 h k or l light chain excretion on urine electrophoresis in the presence of amyloidosis
Minor criteria*	
a.	Bone marrow plasmacytosis 10–30% plasma cells
b.	Monoclonal globulin spike present but < III above
c.	Lytic bone lesions
d.	Residual normal IgM < 50 mg/dl, IgA < 100 mg/dl or IgG < 600 mg/dl
Salmon & Durie staging system	
I	Hb > 10 g/dl; Ca++ normal; bones normal on X-ray or solitary bone plasmacytoma; IgG < 5 g/dl; IgA < 3 g/dl; urine light chain < 4 g/24 h
II	Neither I nor III
III	One or more of Hb < 8.5 g/dl; Ca++ elevated; advanced lytic bone disease; IgG > 7 g/dl; IgA > 5 g/dl; urine light chains > 12 g/24 h
	A Normal renal function
	B Abnormal renal function

*Diagnosis is confirmed with a minimum of 1 major + 1 minor criteria or 3 minor (including a and b).

Making the diagnosis

Signs and symptoms • Anaemia (70% present — normocytic, normochromic)
• Bone pain (60% present) • Renal impairment (50% present) • Fatigue
• Recurrent infections • Reduced height • Hypercalcaemia (30% present)
• Hyperviscosity • Clouded consciousness — headache; blurred vision
• Bleeding diatheses • Osteolytic lesions or pathological fractures
(80% of cases).

Investigations • FBC and ESR (latter normal in 10% of cases) • Blood
chemistry — renal function (see above) • Serum electrophoresis —
paraprotein (pp) band in 80% of cases • Urine electrophoresis — light
chains in 20% with no serum pp; 80% have monoclonal light chains
• Bone marrow > 30% plasma cells diagnostic • Skeletal survey.

Treatment

Chemotherapy Introduced when patient is symptomatic and/or is demonstrated to have progressive disease. Combination of alkylating agent melphalan 10 mg orally daily × 5 and prednisolone 40 mg orally daily × 5. Stopped when pp reaches stability (plateau phase).

High-dose chemotherapy

- Melphalan in doses ≤ 200 mg/m^2 with autologous bone marrow rescue (ABMR).
- Busulphan as a single-agent conditioning agent before bone marrow rescue—less nephrotoxic than melphalan
  — in most cases high-dose methylprednisolone is given with the returned bone marrow to reduce the risk of transfusion of viable myeloma cells with the marrow.
- Bone marrow reconstitution using peripheral blood stem cells harvested following stimulation with haemopoietic growth factors, e.g. granulocyte colony-stimulating factor (GCSF)
  — avoids GA for bone marrow harvest
  — bone marrow recovery reduced from 28 to 14 d
  — protracted neutropenic period reduced.
- Allogeneic bone marrow transplant—recommended only for patients < 60 years of age.
- Interferon-α as single-agent second-line therapy for maintenance of response rates.

Prognosis

- High LDH and B$_2$M (Beta 2 Microglobulin) signify a poor prognosis.
- Melphalan and prednisolone
  — response rate 50%
  — median duration 20 months; median survival 35 months.

Combination chemotherapy has not been shown to be definitely superior despite many randomized studies. The consensus opinion is that combination treatment—vincristine, continuous-infusion adriamycin and high-dose dexamethasone (VAD) or the similar regimen where high-dose methylprednisolone replaces dexamethasone (VAMP)—achieves higher response rates in poor-prognosis myeloma.

- Response rates of almost 80% in both previously treated and untreated patients, with median response durations of 6 and 19 months respectively, were achieved following high-dose chemotherapy with melphalan at 140 mg/m^2 as the 'conditioning regimen'.
- 58% achieved complete remission with 40% survival at 76 months following high-dose therapy with bone marrow rescue.

- Maximum response—50% complete response rate and 80% of patients still in remission at 15 months' follow-up after VAMP chemotherapy followed by melphalan 200 mg/m^2 and ABMR.
- Maintenance with interferon-α
  - 20% response rate as single-agent second-line therapy in myeloma
  - ≤ 39 months' remission post high-dose chemotherapy and ABMR
  - 53% of patients who achieved complete remission were still in remission 4 years after commencement of maintenance interferon-α.

LEUKAEMIA

Leukaemia denotes an uncontrolled growth of the haemopoietic cells in the bone marrow and circulation. The leukaemia may be acute or chronic and involve either the lymphoid or the myeloid series, therefore the four major categories are acute lymphoblastic, acute myeloid, chronic lymphocytic or chronic myeloid. In all leukaemias, the blood cells are less effective than normal and render the patient at risk from infection and/or bleeding.

The *causes* of leukaemia are not known. The *prognosis* differs for the type of leukaemia and the patient's age and will be discussed under each section.

Patients may *present* with lack of energy or dyspnoea (anaemia), infection (low white cell count), mental blunting (very high white cell count, e.g. ALL), joint pains or bruising/bleeding (low platelets or clotting abnormalities). All of these except the high WCC are due to bone marrow failure caused by the leukaemia.

Examination may reveal, in addition to the above, splenomegaly, a swollen thymus gland or enlarged lymph nodes. Occasionally a patient may develop a cranial nerve palsy if the leukaemia involves the CNS. *Diagnosis* is confirmed by bone marrow examination and cytological examination of the CSF. CXR is mandatory.

ACUTE LYMPHOBLASTIC LEUKAEMIA (ALL)

This is the commonest type and accounts for 75% of all childhood leukaemia with 40% of cases developing between 3 and 5 years. In adults, it is relatively rare.

Classification
The French, American, British (FAB) classification denotes three types of ALL—L1, L2, and L3—although it is difficult to differentiate between L1 and L2. A second classification details different sub-types identified by immunological markers (antibodies) against the immature lymphoblasts.

- Common (C) accounts for about 75% of cases. This is commonest in children but all ages may be affected.
- T cell incidence peaks in adolescence. Often the white cell count is very high and is associated with a mediastinal mass on CXR.
- B cell is a rarer tumour and carries a poor prognosis.
- Null cell has no immunological markers.

 The most important prognostic factor is whether the leukaemia is T or B cell since patients with T cell disease (usually older boys with a high presenting white cell count and mediastinal mass) have a worse outlook than does common ALL.

Treatment

Combination chemotherapy initially, to induce remission. Drugs commonly used include methotrexate, vincristine, mercaptopurine and prednisolone. Note that if there is rapid tumour lysis the patient is at risk of renal failure, hyperkalaemia and hyperuricaemia, so a high fluid delivery, allopurinol and regular K^+ checks are necessary. The risk of CNS relapse is reduced by giving prophylactic intrathecal chemotherapy and cranial irradiation. The other so-called sanctuary site is in the testicles. Maintenance chemotherapy is continued for about 2 years.

Intravenous antibiotics, blood transfusions and platelet transfusions are all likely to be required during the treatment period.

Treatment success in ALL is better in children, up to 90% of whom can be cured with combination chemotherapy. In adults aged between 20 and 70 years, this falls to around 30%. Males, black people, high WCC at presentation, CNS involvement and some genetic abnormalities also confer a worse prognosis.

Remission

Confirmed with histological examination of a bone marrow aspirate and biopsy if < 5% of leukaemic blasts can be identified.

High dose chemotherapy with bone marrow transplant is recommended for adults with HLA-matched siblings provided that a remission can be obtained with chemotherapy.

Children with a poor prognosis may also benefit from high dose therapy with bone marrow transplant and studies are currently ongoing.

ACUTE MYELOID LEUKAEMIA (AML)

This is an aggressive form of leukaemia more common in older people and in those who have previously had chemotherapy (e.g. alkylating agents, p. 13).

Classification

There are seven different histological types described in the French-American-British (FAB) classification which describes the appearance of the blast (immature) cells (Table 4.38)

TABLE 4.38 FAB classification of AML	
M1	myeloblastic without maturation
M2	myeloblastic with maturation
M3	hypergranular promyelocytic
M4	myelomonocytic
M5	monocytic or monoblastic
M6	erythroleukaemia (di Gugliemo's syndrome)
M7	acute megakaryoblastic

Making the diagnosis

Similar to ALL. Promyelocytic (M3) leukaemias may present with disseminated intravascular coagulation (DIC).

Treatment

Combination chemotherapy: the main effective drugs include daunorubucin, cytosine arabinoside and thioguanine. The M3 hypergranular promyelocytic leukaemia may have cell differentiation induced by all-trans retinoic acid (ATRA) when treated for 4–6 weeks followed by consolidation with chemotherapy. In addition it is traditional for these patients to have heparin because of the common presentation of DIC.

As in all leukaemias, bone marrow suppression from the tumour and/or the treatment can result in serious infection, bleeding and death.

Maintenance treatment with out-patient cytarabine and 6-thioguanine alternating with daunorubicin did not increase the cure rate of AML and its benefit in prolonging the complete remission rate was marginal, so most centres now give two further courses of combination chemotherapy.

Up to 25% of patients < 60 years are cured with this treatment. Re-treatment at relapse 6 months post treatment is associated with a complete response rate of 50%.

Intensification of treatment
Bone marrow transplant (BMT) is appropriate for many patients who achieve a first remission. Even with this, the overall cure rate for AML is no more than 50%. The quoted fatality rate for patients going through allogeneic BMT is around 30%.

Alternatively, patients may have an autologous BMT with their own marrow being harvested in first remission. The cure rate is not significantly lower than using a donor marrow (allograft), but there is no stimulus to the patient's immune system and this lack of graft-versus-leukaemia effect may be a disadvantage in terms of reducing the quality or duration of the remission. Conversely, the less complicated procedure of autografting carries a lower mortality rate.

Prognosis
Better for patients of lower age, good general fitness, no abnormality in cytogenetics—note that some chromosomal abnormalities are favourable, e.g. t (8;21), t(15;17) — low blast cell count and low LDH and a rapid response to treatment. Treatment results in a complete remission in around 80% of patients aged under 60 years.

CHRONIC MYELOID LEUKAEMIA

Making the diagnosis
Chronic myeloid or granulocytic leukaemia (CML/CGL) may be diagnosed on a routine blood count where a raised mature white cell count is identified. Some centres differentiate between the two and define CGL as the entity of marked splenomegaly with high WCC. Dividing cells have a Philadelphia chromosome — translocation of genetic material between the long arms of chromosome 9 and 22.

Patients may initially be totally asymptomatic in a 'stable' or 'chronic' phase. Treatment at this stage shrinks the spleen and reduces the WCC.

At around 4 years later, the 'accelerated', 'blastic' or acute transformation phase may develop and in 20% of cases it is the lymphoid rather than the myeloid cells which transform to result in fever, increased splenomegaly, rising WCC and weight loss. Occasionally, patients may simply develop a myelofibrosis.

Treatment
Chemotherapy has changed from traditional alkylating agents busulphan and hydroxyurea to interferon alpha (IFNα). Daily treatment with 9 mega-units results in rapid resolution of symptoms and signs in the majority of patients (70% CR), and reversal of the Ph+ chromosome may be seen in 65% of patients. These patients have a better survival rate than those who remain Ph+.

Hydroxyurea remains the drug of second choice. Busulphan is still used in older patients because of the lack of importance of infertility in that group.

In the accelerated phase, palliative chemotherapy similar to an AML regimen may be helpful, but the effect is normally short-lived. In the event of a lymphoid transformation patients may benefit from ALL type of regimens. The reinduction of the chronic phase can then be maintained for several months with use of craniospinal or intrathecal treatments.

Bone marrow transplant in chronic phase For patients < 55 who have an HLA-matched or near-matched sibling, this can achieve 4-year survival rates of 70%, although only 15% of these are relapse-free. At relapse, 80% of patients will re-enter remission on infusion of lymphoid cells from the original donor.

Radiotherapy Effective in CML but it has now been superseded by chemotherapy except where there is enormous splenomegaly or painful bone metastases. Craniospinal irradiation can be effective in CNS disease.

Prognosis
With these novel approaches prognosis from diagnosis has improved so that median survival is now around 5 years. Significant splenomegaly, high leucocyte or platelet count and anaemia are all associated with a worse outlook.

CHRONIC LYMPHOCYTIC LEUKAEMIA (CLL)
This most common of the chronic lymphoid leukaemias is caused by uncontrolled proliferation of mature B lymphocytes.

Making the diagnosis
It may present with recurrent infection, lymphadenopathy or abdominal discomfort due to splenomegaly or hepatomegaly. The diagnosis is suggested by the FBC and bone marrow aspirate and trephine will confirm. The Biner staging system is detailed in Table 4.39.

TABLE 4.39 CLL: Biner staging system	
A	No anaemia or thrombocytopenia; fewer than 3 lymph node areas involved
B	No anaemia or thrombocytopenia; three or more lymph node areas involved
C	Anaemia and/or thrombocytopenia with any number of nodal sites involved

Treatment

Determined by the stage of disease and the patient's symptoms. If there is a stable high WCC and no evidence of bone marrow failure or haemolysis, the patient may be observed for a number of years. First line management is now with chlorambucil with or without prednisolone, which is an easy, non-toxic out-patient therapy. Some patients develop an overt haemolytic anaemia and this will respond to steroid therapy.

With repeated, intermittent courses of chemotherapy, the CLL may become resistant and there are now several second-line effective agents (fludarabine, 2-chlorodeoxyadenosine) which may well supersede chlorambucil in the future. Response rates in previously treated patients are around 60% with either drug.

Irradiation of bulky nodal sites or spleen can be effective in patients who are unfit for or non-compliant with chemotherapy, and for those who develop chemoresistant disease.

Prognosis

Prognosis depends on the rate of progression of the disease, but because it is most common in elderly patients, other illnesses may often be the cause of death while the CLL is in a plateau phase.

AIDS-RELATED CANCER

More than 40% of people with AIDS are diagnosed as having a malignant disease at some time during their illness. The risk increases as survival with the disease is prolonged. Development of a particular malignancy may be an 'AIDS-defining event' in patients with HIV infection. Those defining tumours are:

- Kaposi's sarcoma
- non-Hodgkin's lymphoma
- cervical cancer.

KAPOSI'S SARCOMA

More advanced HIV infection is associated with KS, which can be a very aggressive disease in this setting. Exogenous steroids may stimulate development of KS and their withdrawal can cause regression of the lesions.

Risk factors
- Genetic predisposition.
- More common in HIV-infected homosexual or bisexual men (incidence 18%).
- Other groups with HIV infection (incidence around 5%).

Making the diagnosis
- Tumour usually develops on skin or mucous membranes, less commonly in the viscera.
- Purple, subepidermal, vascular lesion composed of spindle cells and mononuclear cell infiltrates.

Treatment
Dictated by the number and site of lesions and by the patient's immunological status. The CD4 lymphocyte count ($> 200/mm^3$) and bone marrow function are most important.

- < 25 mucocutaneous lesions: observation only, with local irradiation when necessary
- CD4 count $> 400/mm^3$: response to interferon-α is 70% and is proportional to the count
- More advanced and visceral KS: systemic chemotherapy with single agent or combination vinca alkaloids, etoposide, doxorubicin and bleomycin the most active agents achieves response rates of 30–60%.

Maintenance with interferon-α may be commenced on completion of chemotherapy.

Prognosis

Advanced pulmonary KS is associated with a survival of < 6 months.

NHL

The incidence of NHL in people with AIDS is 4–10% and increases with prolonged survival. The disease is widely disseminated at diagnosis, has a higher than usual incidence of CNS and other extranodal involvement, is of intermediate or high-grade histology and is aggressive.

The majority of AIDS NHLs are B-cell tumours, but there is no evidence that HIV is the transforming agent. EBV, present in 50% of samples, is more likely to be the infective agent responsible for neoplastic transformation of the B cells.

Treatment

Should be most aggressive in patients with good prognostic features. Early introduction of gCSF will allow delivery of optimal chemotherapy doses without causing severe marrow toxicity.

Prognosis

Good prognostic features include: • higher performance status • stage I or II disease • no bone marrow involvement • non-immunoblastic histology • no B symptoms • no previous AIDS-defining events • CD4 count > 100/mm^3.

Median survival: 6 months

Median survival for patients who achieve a complete response (approximately 60%): 15 months

OTHER TUMOURS

- Basal cell carcinoma of the skin
  — risk > 18 times greater in HIV-infected haemophilic men.
- Hodgkin's disease
  — often presents at an advanced, symptomatic stage
  — mixed cellularity histological type
  — shorter survival time despite treatment.

CARCINOMA OF UNKNOWN PRIMARY SITE

Cancers of unknown primary site (CUPS) account for up to 9% of neoplasms. Common sites of presentation include nodes, liver, bone and lung. There may be a single affected node with no evident source of the tumour even after biopsy, and no evidence of residual tumour once the node is removed. Usually there is widespread metastatic disease. Patients with tumours categorized as 'poorly differentiated or undifferentiated neoplasm' form an important subgroup: a proportion of them will have a NHL which may be curable with the correct chemotherapy.

Histology (→ Table 4.40)

TABLE 4.40 CUPS: histology		
Estimation of tumour types based on retrospective studies		
Adenocarcinoma		60%
	Specific subgroup 6%	
	Nonspecific 54%	
Poorly differentiated carcinoma		30%
	Lymphoma, melanoma, sarcoma 3%	
	Specific carcinoma 1%	
	Nonidentified 26%	
Poorly differentiated malignant neoplasm		5%
	Lymphoma 3%	
	Melanoma, sarcoma, other 1%	
	Nonidentified 1%	
SCC		5%
	Specific subgroup 4%	
	Nonspecific 1%	

Making the diagnosis

Signs and symptoms Symptoms relate to the extent of tumour, e.g. fatigue and pain.

Investigations • Full history and clinical examination, including pelvis, rectum, nasopharyngeal space (for SCC cervical node) • FBC and chemistry • CXR • CT scan chest, abdomen and pelvis • Adequate biopsy of malignant tissue (not simply FNA) with immunohistochemistry — chromosomal analysis in biopsies which evade other categorization — chromosomal abnormalities may be specific to some lymphomas or to germ cell tumours • Mammogram

in women > 45 years • Endoscopy and colonoscopy (adenocarcinoma)
• Tumour markers. **NB**: with the exception of PSA, may give an indication of possible primary site but rarely definitive:

— PSA
— CEA (lung/colon)
— CA125 (80% of ovarian tumours)
— bHCG (germ cell)
— AFP (germ cell/hepatocellular carcinoma)
— CA19.9 (pancreas).

Treatment

Unfit or elderly patients

Since there is no prospect of cure, the option to treat with symptomatic measures only should be discussed with the patient—radiotherapy to painful bone metastases, steroids to improve a sense of well-being and appetite, analgesics, etc. However, postmenopausal women with adenocarcinoma may respond to tamoxifen (non-toxic) if the occult primary tumour originates in the breast.

Fit patients who want treatment

The patient must be given a full explanation of the situation and prognosis. Management options include:

• Observation until symptoms develop
• Early intervention with platinum-based chemotherapy
• Entry into a Phase I drug study if 'best guess' therapy is unsuccessful.

Non-SCC The commonest tumours are lung, colon, prostate and breast. On this basis platinum and 5-fluorouracil are appropriate 'best guess' drugs to include in a regimen. In women this would also be effective in 60% of ovarian or peritoneal adenocarcinomas.

• Axillary nodes may arise from an occult breast primary. A logical approach is systemic chemotherapy (high risk of distant metastases) and tamoxifen, with axillary clearance for control of nodal disease.
• A trial of hormone therapy for prostate cancer may be successful.

> ⚠ If patients have not responded after 2 cycles of platinum-containing chemotherapy, it should be discontinued. Most centres would advocate 6 cycles of chemotherapy in total. Consolidation of response with high-dose chemotherapy is rarely appropriate.

SCC

Neck nodes May respond well to radical neck dissection ± radiotherapy, with up to 50% 5-year survival.

Inguinal nodes May arise from anal carcinoma. Locoregional surgery ± postoperative radiotherapy may be curative.

Prognosis
Survival is significantly improved in patients who respond to treatment. Overall: median survival 4 months.

MALIGNANT NECK NODE

Patients presenting with a malignant lymph node in the neck from an unknown primary should be managed as follows:

Clinical examination
- Scalp, face, neck, upper chest wall, lips, tongue, palate, buccal mucosa, thyroid.
- ENT examination of nasopharynx, oropharynx, hypopharynx, larynx.
- Chest (? Pancoast's tumour).
- Abdomen (? Virchow's node).
- Testes (? testicular tumour).
- Prostate.
- Other lymph node sites (? lymphoma).

FNAC of lymph node Diagnosis of melanoma or carcinoma is usually possible, proceeding to needle core biopsy if more tissue is required. If lymphoma is suspected, proceed to

Open biopsy Avoid in patients who may require a radical neck dissection, so as not to compromise the surgical field and incisions. It is usually reserved for a clinical diagnosis of lymphoma.

'Hunt the primary' These tests are determined by the results of the above.
- SCC—CXR, bronchoscopy, EUA, 'blind' biopsy of nasopharynx.
- Adenocarcinoma—gastroscopy, abdominal ultrasound, abdominal CT, colonoscopy, laparoscopy.
- Melanoma—may have a regressed primary, but look for other metastases on CXR, liver ultrasound.
- Lymphoma—staging (see p. 150).
- Tumour marker analysis.

APPENDICES

COMMONLY USED CHEMOTHERAPY AGENTS

Drug	Tumour	Side-effect	Metabolism/administration
Alkylating agents			
Cyclophosphamide	CLL NHL and Hodgkin's disease Breast cancer	Haemorrhagic cystitis (ensure hydration and MESNA with higher doses) Alopecia Bone marrow suppression (platelets spared) Mucositis Cardiac toxicity	*Metabolism*: hepatic to active metabolite; peak activity 2–3 hours post intravenous (IV) injection. *Administration*: oral dosing: 50 mg daily. IV injections up to 2 g/m^2 by 24 hour infusion
Ifosfamide	Lymphomas Sarcoma Lung cancer Cervix	Haemorrhagic cystitis Bone marrow suppression Alopecia Encephalopathy (increased risk if low albumin, poor renal function) Nausea and vomiting	*Metabolism*: similar to cyclophosphamide. *Administration*: IV infusion 1.5–2.5 g/m^2 daily for 3–5 days
Melphalan	Multiple myeloma Ovary Sarcoma Breast	Bone marrow suppression Alopecia } high Nausea and vom. } doses	*Administration*: orally 2–10 mg daily. IV 1 mg/kg 4–6 weekly.
Chlorambucil	CLL Lymphomas Ovary Waldenstrom's macroglobulinaemia	Bone marrow suppression	*Administration*: orally 2–10 mg daily.

Drug	Tumour	Side-effect	Metabolism/administration
Antimetabolites			
Methotrexate (MTX)	Acute leukaemia Choriocarcinoma Squamous cell carcinoma	Myelosuppression Mucositis Pneumonitis } with Intestinal haem. } high Renal toxicity } doses Cirrhosis Chronic demyelination } IT adminis- Arachnoiditis } tration only	*Metabolism:* largely excreted unchanged in the urine therefore measurement of renal function is mandatory; folinic acid given orally or intravenously from 24 hours post commencement of the MTX will inhibit its action and 'rescue' the patient from excessive toxicity; duration of rescue is determined from serial plasma level measurement; distribution of MTX into the 'third space', e.g. ascitic or pleural fluid will increase the risk of delayed toxicity as the drug is released into the circulation, therefore these should be drained or rescue should be prolonged in this situation. *Administration:* orally 2.5 mg daily. IV up to 5 g by continuous infusion. Intrathecally (IT) as prophylaxis against or treatment of central nervous system involvement, especially in leukaemias and lymphomas at a dose of up to 15 mg.
5-fluorouracil (5-FU)	Stomach Colon Breast Head and neck	Mucositis Plantar palmar syndrome Bone marrow suppression Cardiac ataxia	*Administration:* oral delivery has been superseded by IV administration, and continuous infusion therapy up to 300 mg/m² daily is both less toxic and more effective than bolus dosing. Oral pyridoxine 200 mg × 3 daily can prevent the plantar palmar syndrome.
Cytosine arabinoside (ARA-C)	Acute leukaemia (AML)	Myelosuppression Nausea and vomiting Diarrhoea Mucositis Hepatic dysfunction	*Administration:* scheduling is important and continuous infusion or 8-hourly bolus doses at 100 mg/m² are more effective than once daily injections.

Drug	Tumour	Side-effect	Metabolism/administration
Antimetabolites			
6-Mercaptopurine (6-MP)	Acute leukaemia (ALL)	Myelosuppression Hepatic dysfunction Renal failure (from hyperuricaemia)	*Metabolism*: xanthine oxidase is a vital enzyme in 6-MP metabolism. Allopurinol given to reduce uric acid levels in patients whose tumour may undergo rapid breakdown inhibits xanthine oxidase, therefore concurrent administration of these drugs will result in increased toxicity unless the 6-MP dose is reduced by up to 70%. *Administration*: orally 50–100 mg/m² daily.
6-Thioguanine (6-TG)	Myeloid leukaemia	Bone marrow suppression Mucositis Diarrhoea Hepatic dysfunction	*Administration*: orally 2–2.5 mg/kg daily
Vinca alkaloids			
Vincristine	Leukaemia Lymphoma	Neuropathy —sensory —motor Constipation Alopecia Convulsions } less SIADH } commonly Visual upset	*Administration*: IV injection is limited to doses of 2 mg max (1–1.4 mg/m²) with prompt reduction in dose if there is evidence of neuropathy.
Vinblastine	Hodgkin's lymphoma	Myelosuppression Vesicant if extravasated mucositis Alopecia Neurotoxicity—rarely	*Administration*: IV injection up to 6 mg/m².
Vindesine	Malignant melanoma	Leucopenia Mild sensory neuropathy	*Administration*: IV injection 3 mg/m² weekly.

Drug	Tumour	Side-effect	Metabolism/administration
Antimitotic antibiotics			
Daunorubicin	Leukaemia	Nausea and vomiting Bone marrow supp. Cardiotoxicity Acute—arrhythmia, LVF, Chronic—myopathy Alopecia	*Administration:* 40–60 mg/m^2 on alternate days up to 3 injections
Doxorubicin	Breast Bronchogenic Sarcoma Ovary Gastric	As above; a total dose of > 550 mg/m^2 results in cardiac failure in ~10% patients; risk↑ with age, previous RT	*Administration:* IV 20–120 mg/m^2 1–3 weekly; infusional therapy is also effective
Epirubicin	Breast Gastric Sarcoma Bronchogenic	As above but less GI and cardiac toxicity	*Administration:* IV injection 20–80 mg/m^2 3 weekly. Non-anthracycline antibiotics act in the same ways as the anthracyclines described above
Actinomycin-D	Paediatric tumours Choriocarcinoma Soft tissue sarcoma Testicular teratoma	Myelosuppression Nausea and vomiting Diarrhoea Mucositis Radiation recall Vesicant	*Administration:* IV injection 10–15 μg/kg daily for 4 days, 3–4 weekly
Mitomycin C	Breast Bladder	Myelosuppression (delayed) Nausea and vomiting Diarrhoea Renal failure (> 100 mg cumulative) Pulmonary infiltration/fibrosis Vesicant	*Administration:* IV injection up to 10 mg weekly; intravesical instillation is possible for bladder cancer

Drug	Tumour	Side-effect	Metabolism/administration
Antimitotic antibiotics			
Bleomycin	Testicular teratoma Lymphomas Squamous cell carcinomas	Pneumonitis-fibrosis (> 300 mg cumulative; increased risk if prev. lung damage) Skin changes (50% pts) Fevers	*Administration:* IV injection 2–90 mg; intrapleural instillation via a chest drain for pleurodesis 60 mg stat.
Non-classical alkylating agents			
Cisplatin	Testicular teratoma Ovary Bladder Head and neck Breast Lung	Nausea and vomiting Neuropathy Deafness Tinnitus Renal failure Mild bone marrow supp. Gastric hypomagnesaemia Hypokalaemia	*Administration:* IV 50–120 mg/m² daily (or 20 mg/m² daily × 5 days) following hydration and mannitol; posthydration also necessary (total approx. 3 litres), 3–4 weekly cycle. **NB**: check renal function on alternate courses
Carboplatin	as above	Less nausea and vomiting Thrombocytopenia	*Administration:* IV 400–1000 mg/m² or better AUC6–12 according to Calvert's formula using EDTA (see below). Monthly treatment
Dacarbazine (DTIC)	Melanoma Sarcoma Hodgkin's	Nausea and vomiting Bone marrow supp. Alopecia Liver enzyme upset	A purine analogue which may, following metabolism, act like an alkylating agent *Administration:* IV 250–400 mg/m² 3 weekly
Procarbazine			An analogue of the monoamine oxidase inhibitors. It may act by alkylation

Drug	Tumour	Side-effect	Metabolism/administration
Non-classical alkylating agents			
Procarbazine	Hodgkin's	Nausea and vomiting Bone marrow supp. Somnolence Confusion Ataxia	*Administration:* orally 50–300 mg/day 3-weekly
Anthracenediones			
Mitozantrone	Breast Lymphomas	Bone marrow supp. Nausea and vomiting Alopecia	*Administration:* IV 10–14 mg/m² 4–6-weekly
Epidophyllotoxins			
Etoposide	Lung (small cell) Testicular teratoma	Bone marrow suppression Alopecia Nausea Periph. neurop. (mild) Liver enzyme upset	*Metabolism:* partially renal so toxicity may be worse with impaired renal function *Administration:* IV up to 120 mg/m² × 5 days every 3 weeks; oral up to 300 mg/m² daily × 5 every 3 weeks
Taxanes			
Taxol	Ovary Breast	Alopecia Neutropenia Neuropathy	*Administration:* IV up to 390 mg/m² in 24 hours 3-weekly

Calvert's Formula
Total dose of carboplatin = (creatinine clearance + 25) × AUC (Area Under Curve desired). For example, with a creatinine clearance of 60 ml/min and a desired AUC of 6, the total dose of carboplatin is (60 + 25) × 6, i.e. 510 mg.

WHO PERFORMANCE SCALE

0: Able to carry out all normal activity without restriction.
1: Restricted in physically strenuous activity, but ambulatory and able to carry out light work.
2: Ambulatory and capable of all self-care, but unable to carry out work; up and about more than 50% of waking hours.
3: Capable only of limited self-care; confined to bed more than 50% of waking hours.
4: Completely disabled; cannot carry out any self-care; totally confined to bed or chair.

COMMON TOXICITY CRITERIA

Grade	0	1	2	3	4
Gastrointestinal					
Nausea	None	Able to eat—reasonable intake	Intake significantly decreased but can eat	No significant intake	—
Vomiting	None	One episode in 24 hours	2–5 episodes in 24 hours	6–10 episodes in 24 hours	>10 episodes in 24 hours or requiring parenteral support
Diarrhoea	None	Increase of 2–3 stools/day over pre-Rx	Increase of 4–6 stools/day or nocturnal stools, or moderate cramping	Increase of 7–9 stools/day or incontinence or severe cramping	Increase of 3–10 stools/day or grossly bloody diarrhoea, or need for parenteral support
Stomatitis	None	Painless ulcers, erythema, or mild soreness	Painful erythema, oedema, or ulcers, but can eat	Painful erythema, oedema, or ulcers and cannot eat	Requires parenteral or or enteral support
Dermatological					
Skin	None or no change	Scattered macular or papular eruption or erythema that is asymptomatic	Scattered macular or papular eruption or erythema with pruritus or other associated symptoms	Generalised symptomatic macular, papular, or vesicular eruption	Exfoliative dermatitis or ulcerating dermetitis

Grade	0	1	2	3	4
Neurological					
Neuro-sensory	None or no change	Mild paraesthesia, loss of deep tendon reflexes	Mild or moderate objective sensory loss; moderate paraesthesia	Severe objective sensory loss or paraesthesia interfering with functioning	—
Neuro-motor	None or no change	Subjective weakness; no objective findings	Mild objective weakness without significant impairment	Objective weakness with impairment of function	Paralysis
Neuro-cortical	None	Mild somnolence or agitation	Moderate somnolence or agitation	Severe somnolence, agitation, confusion, disorientation or hallucinations	Coma, seizures, toxic psychosis
Neuro-cerebellar	None	Slight incoordin., dysdiadochokinesis	Intention tremor, dysmetria, slurred speech, nystagmus	Locomotor ataxia	Cerebellar necrosis
Neuro-mood	No change	Mild anxiety or depression	Moderate anxiety or depression	Severe anxiety or depression	Suicidal ideation
Neuro-headache	None	Mild	Moderate or severe but transient	Unrelenting and severe	—
Neuro-constipation	None or no change	Mild	Moderate	Severe	Ileus
Neuro-hearing	None or no change	Asymptom., hearing loss audiometry only	Tinnitus	Hearing loss interfering with function, correctable with hearing aid	Deafness not correctable

Grade	0	1	2	3	4
Neurological					
Neuro-vision	None or no change	—	—	Symptomatic blindness subtotal loss of vision	
Pain	None	Mild	Moderate	Severe	Intolerable
Behavioural change	None	Change, not disruptive to family	Disruptive to patient or family	Harmful to others or self	Psychotic behaviour
Dizziness/vertigo	None	Non-disabling	—	Disabling	—
Taste	Normal	Slightly altered taste, metallic taste	Markedly altered taste		
Insomnia	Normal	Occasional difficulty sleeping, may need pills		Difficulty sleeping despite medication	
Neurologic—other	Normal	Mild	Moderate	Severe	Life-threatening
Haematologic					
WBC	≥4.0	3.0–3.9	2.0–2.9	1.0–1.9	<1.0
Platelets	Normal	75.0–normal	50.0–74.9	25.0–49.9	<25.0
Hgb g/100 ml	Normal	10.0–normal	8.0–10.0	6.5–7.9	<6.5
g/L	Normal	100–normal	80–100	65–79	<65
mmol/L	Normal	6.2–normal	4.95–6.2	4.0–4.9	<4.0
Granulocytes/bands	≥2.0	1.5–1.9	1.0–1.4	0.5–0.9	<0.5
Lymphocytes	≥2.0	1.5–1.9	1.0–1.4	0.5–0.9	<0.5
Haematologic—other	None	Mild	Moderate	Severe	Life-threatening

Data from the National Cancer Institute

CRITERIA OF RESPONSE

RESPONSE EVALUATION (WHO)

Complete response (CR)—resolution of all measurable or evaluable disease.

Partial response (PR)—greater than or equal to 50% reduction in measurable or evaluable disease in the absence of progression in any particular disease site.

Stable disease (NC or SD)—less than 50% decrease or less than 25% increase in measurable or evaluable disease.

Progressive disease (PD)—greater than 25% increase in measurable or evaluable disease or development of a new lesion.

SURFACE AREA NOMOGRAM

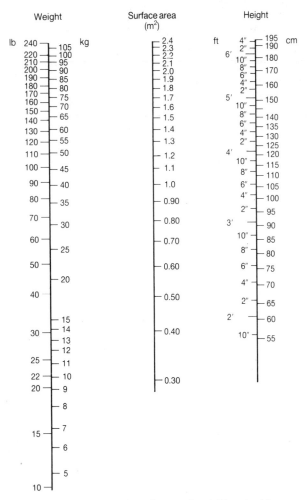

Fig. 5.1 A nomogram for surface area from height and weight.

DERMATOMAL ANATOMY

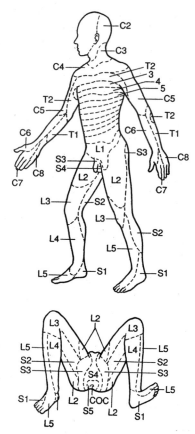

Fig. 5.2 Dermatomal anatomy.

DRUG DEVELOPMENT AND CLINICAL TRIALS

The early investigation of a novel anticancer drug in man is the Phase I trial, and the starting dose is normally one tenth of the murine MTD. The patients may be people whose cancer has been extensively pretreated with conventional agents which have become ineffective, or they may have a tumour for which there is no useful conventional treatment (e.g. mesothelioma). In all cases it is imperative that the patients in a Phase I trial fulfil basic fitness criteria and are able to give fully informed consent prior to receipt of the new drug. This is especially important since the aim of a Phase I trial is to establish the toxicity profile of the drug, to investigate the body's handling of it (pharmacokinetics) and to find the maximum tolerated dose. The latter is established through a carefully controlled increase in the dose delivered. The response rate in Phase I trials is in the order of 7%. In some cases the scheduling of the drug will also be investigated in the Phase I trial, for example to see whether there is evidence of alteration in toxicity or efficacy depending on whether the drug is given once weekly or daily × 5.

Provided that the new drug has an acceptable toxicity profile, it will move on to Phase II trials. Here the aim is to establish the efficacy of the drug in treatment of specific tumours. Again the patients will probably have received previous chemotherapies to which their tumours are or have become resistant. The starting dose for Phase II trials is selected from the data obtained from the Phase I trials, and different schedules may again be studied. Finally, if the Phase II trial indicates that the drug is a useful anticancer agent, it will be tested in a randomised trial against the best available (conventional) treatment for a particular tumour in a Phase III trial.

Clinical Trials — from drug development to use in vivo

Phase I
Aims To establish the human toxicity of a new drug through delivering carefully selected increasing doses to patients; to establish the safe dose at which to start further trials with the drug; to measure the body's handling (pharmacokinetics) of the drug.

Included Consenting patients with histologically proven cancer who are fit and who may have received previous conventional chemotherapy and failed to respond or responded and relapsed. In tumours where there is no effective conventional treatment, eg. mesothelioma, pancreatic cancer, direct entry to a Phase I trial may be appropriate. The starting dose is usually 10% of the dose found to be lethal in 10% (LD10) of animals treated in the preclinical studies. Note that no measurable responses are expected in a Phase I trial.

Clinical Trials — from drug development to use in vivo *(continued)*

Phase II
Aims To establish the antitumour activity of the drug against a particular tumour type in a patient population where no curative therapy is possible; to obtain further information on the drug's toxicity.

Included Consenting patients who may not have had previous anticancer therapy. If there is no standard therapy for the tumour, the new drug may be randomised against a 'best supportive care' treatment option, but Phase II studies are normally unrandomised.

Phase III
Aims To compare the new drug with conventional best therapy. Included: If antitumour activity is established in Phase II trials the drug is then compared with the standard therapy in a prospective, randomised controlled trial. If the tumour is normally treated with combination therapy (e.g. lymphoma), the new drug will be incorporated into one arm of the study only. Large numbers of consenting patients should be included.

Phase IV
Aims To establish efficacy of drugs in adjuvant trials; to determine long-term toxicity of therapy.

INCIDENCE AND RISK

TABLE Estimates of the % of cohort who develop cancer over a lifetime, and the lifetime risk*

Males	%	Risk
Lung	9.1	1 in 11
Skin (non-melanoma)	5.7	1 in 18
Prostate	4.4	1 in 23
Bladder	2.8	1 in 35
Colon	2.6	1 in 38
Stomach	2.4	1 in 42
Rectum	2.0	1 in 50
NHL	1.1	1 in 93
Pancreas	1.1	1 in 95
Oesophagus	1.0	1 in 96

Females	%	Risk
Breast	8.6	1 in 12
Skin (non-melanoma)	5.0	1 in 20
Lung	3.8	1 in 26
Colon	3.1	1 in 33
Ovary	1.8	1 in 55
Rectum	1.5	1 in 67
Cervix	1.4	1 in 72
Stomach	1.4	1 in 72
Uterus	1.3	1 in 75
Bladder	1.1	1 in 93

* Reproduced by permission of the Cancer Research Campaign

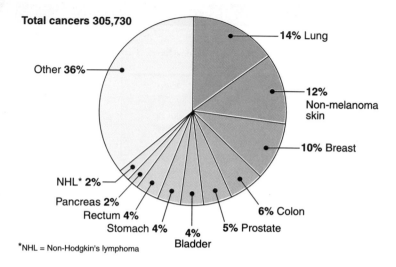

Total cancers 305,730

Other **36%**

14% Lung

12% Non-melanoma skin

10% Breast

6% Colon

5% Prostate

4% Bladder

Stomach **4%**

Rectum **4%**

Pancreas **2%**

NHL* **2%**

*NHL = Non-Hodgkin's lymphoma

Fig. 5.3 Ten most common cancers, UK 1988. Reproduced by permission of the Cancer Research Campaign.

INDEX

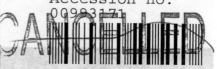

CONTENTS

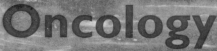

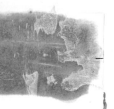

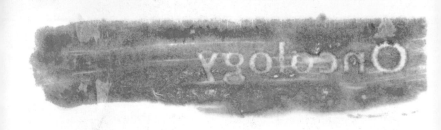

For Churchill Livingstone:

Publisher: Laurence Hunter
Project editor: Jim Killgore
Copy editor: Alison Bowers
Project controller: Kay Hunston
Design direction: Erik Bigland
Page layout: Kate Walshaw